A Textbook of Pharmaceutical Quality Assurance

A Textbook of Pharmaceutical Quality Assurance

Prof. K. P. R. Chowdary

Former Principal
A. U. College of Pharmaceutical Sciences, Andhra University
Visakhapatnam, A. P.

and

Research Director
Vikas Institute of Pharmaceutical Sciences
Rajahmundry, A. P.

PharmaMed Press

An imprint of Pharma Book Syndicate

A unit of BSP Books Pvt. Ltd.

4-4-309/316, Giriraj Lane,
Sultan Bazar, Hyderabad - 500 095.

A Textbook of Pharmaceutical Quality Assurance ***by***
Prof. K. P. R. Chowdary

Published by

PharmaMed Press

An imprint of Pharma Book Syndicate

A unit of BSP Books Pvt. Ltd.

4-4-309/316, Giriraj Lane, Sultan Bazar, Hyderabad - 500 095.
Phone: 040-23445688, 23445600; Fax: 91+40-23445611
E-mail: info@pharmamedpress.com
www.pharmamedpress.com/pharmamedpress.net

Printed at

Aditya Offset Process (I) Pvt. Ltd.
Hyderabad.

ISBN: 978-93-89354-96-6

Dedicated to

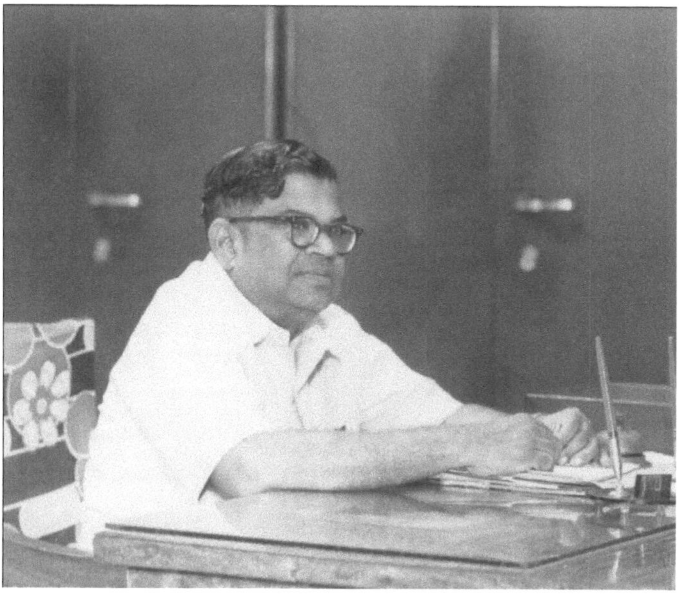

My Teacher, Guide and Well Wisher
Prof.V. SUBBA RAO
(1920-1990)

THE INDIAN PHARMACEUTICAL ASSOCIATION
Kalina, Santacruz (East), Mumbai – 400098, India.

FOREWORD

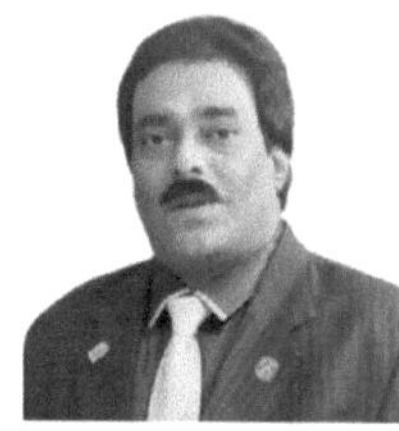

I am extremely happy and delighted to write the foreward to a textbook written by one of the senior most professors of pharmacy in the country. This textbook on Pharmaceutical Quality Assurance is a unique attempt, which fulfilled all the requirements of the students, teachers and industry professionals to acquire a comprehensive and updated knowledge of all aspects of Pharmaceutical quality assurance. The book covers the entire syllabus prescribed by Pharmacy Council of India (PCI) for the subject of Pharmaceutical quality assurance in B. Pharm and M. Pharm programs under revised uniform regulations introduced in 2017. I am sure that this book will be of immense use as ready reckoner and strongly recommend to pharmacy students and as well the teachers of B. Pharm, M. Pharm and Pharm.D.

I being the President of IPA, Mumbai and expert member of the PCI syllabus committee congratulate the author for his commendable efforts and wish him to bring out many more books in his area of expertise i.e. Pharmaceutical Quality Assurance and Pharmaceutical Technology in future.

With Best Wishes.

President, IPA

FOREWORD

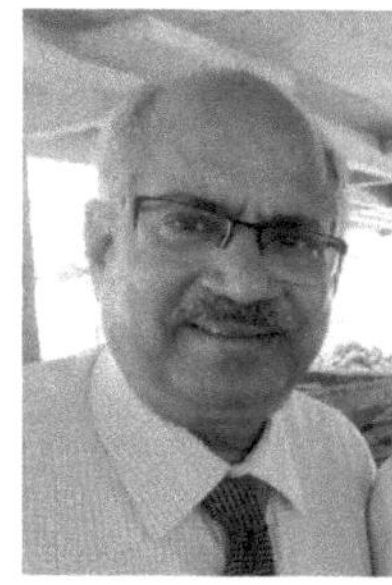

It gives me great pleasure to pen a foreword for the book entitled "A Textbook of Pharmaceutical Quality Assurance" authored by Prof. K. P. R. Chowdary. This book is expected to meet the curricular requirements of the course, pharmaceutical quality assurance included in the syllabus prescribed by the Pharmacy Council of India for B. Pharm and M. Pharm courses. It has long been observed that the B. Pharm and M. Pharm courses in India fail to meet the requirements and expectations of Pharmaceutical industry since the curricular content does not address issues that are critical to the functioning of the pharmaceutical industry. In a bid to bridge this gap, the Pharmacy Council of India revised B. Pharm and M. Pharm syllabi and introduced courses that would enhance the understanding of fresh graduates about industrial operations. Nevertheless, a course on quality assurance would still have not made much difference due to the unavailability of a concise reference textbook for students. Such a lacuna has now been fulfilled by this textbook of Pharmaceutical Quality Assurance, which provides in a nutshell basic information needed to understand concepts related to quality assurance such as total quality management, good manufacturing and good laboratory practices, calibration and validation of analytical equipment, ICH guidelines, ISO certifications and materials management including packaging materials. Absence of such a comprehensive textbook would have made the students refer to several lengthy and complicated resources available on the internet to gain a basic understanding of these concepts. This textbook of Pharmaceutical Quality Assurance will prove to be just right for the students taking Pharmaceutical Quality Assurance course.

Rao V. S. V. Vadlamudi, Ph.D.,

May 1, 2019,
Hyderabad

PREFACE

In the light of globalization and global marketing of pharmaceutical products the concept of 'Quality' as becomes a key factor for the success of pharmaceutical industry. A large number of concepts, guidelines, regulations and practices were developed globally by various organizations and governmental bodies that have concern over quality. The drug regulating authorities globally and local governments provided guidelines and regulations to produce quality products. In this context quality assurance and quality management has become a specialized area of study that deals with the practices to be adopted in pharmaceutical industry to produce quality products. Voluminous literature has accumulated in this area making difficult for the industrial pharmacists and UG and PG students of pharmacy to acquire good knowledge of the subject. The Pharmacy Council of India, New Delhi has also introduced courses on pharmaceutical quality assurance in the revised uniform syllabus prescribed for B Pharm and M Pharm courses. This textbook deals with all aspects of pharmaceutical quality assurance needed for an industrial pharmacist and the book covers the entire syllabus prescribed by PCI for the subject of pharmaceutical quality assurance in B Pharm and M Pharm programs. The author has 40 years of experience in teaching pharmaceutical quality assurance, pharmaceutical management and related subjects at UG and PG level in Andhra University, Visakhapatnam and other pharmacy institutions, which helped him in writing this textbook in simple, easily understandable form.

The key assests of the book include; (i) The book provides a comprehensive knowledge of various aspects of Pharmaceutical Quality assurance as per Industry needs. (ii) The book covers the entire syllabus prescribed for the subject by Pharmacy Council of India, New Delhi for UG and PG programs. (iii) Huge information on the subject is presented in condensed and cohesive form. (iv) The subject is presented in simple easily understandable in logical flow for the purpose of Pharmacy UG and PG students. (v) Current updated guidelines and regulations related to drug development, manufacture and supply are included. As such the book provides latest knowledge on the subject.

Prof. K. P. R. Chowdary

CONTENTS

CHAPTER 4

ICH STABILITY TESTING GUIDELINES AND PROCEUDURES

CHAPTER 5

QUALITY BY DESIGN (QbD)

CHAPTER 8

GOOD MANUFACTURING PRACTICES (GMP) - Part 1 (Introduction, Summary, Organization, Personnel and Premises)

CHAPTER 9

GOOD MANUFACTURING PRACTICES (GMP) - Part II (Equipment and Raw Materials)

CHPATER - 1

Quality Assurance, Quality Management and GMP

Learning Objectives

To learn about definitions and concepts of

- Quality
- Quality Assurance
- Quality Management
- Elements of Quality Management
- Quality Control
- Comparison of Quality Assurance and Quality Control
- Principles of GMP

Quality Management

In the drug industry at large, quality management is usually defined as the aspect of management function that determines and implements the "quality policy", i.e., the overall intention and direction of an organization regarding quality, as formally expressed and authorized by top management.

The basic elements of quality management are:

- an appropriate infrastructure or "quality system", encompassing the organizational structure, procedures, processes and resources;
- systematic actions necessary to ensure adequate confidence that a product (or service) will satisfy given requirements for quality. The totality of these actions is termed "quality assurance".

Within an organization, quality assurance serves as a management tool. In contractual situations, quality assurance also serves to generate confidence in the supplier.

The concepts of quality assurance, GMP and quality control are interrelated aspects of quality management. They are described here in order to emphasize their relationship and their fundamental importance to the production and control of pharmaceutical products.

Quality Assurance

Principle: "Quality assurance" is a wide-ranging concept covering all matters that individually or collectively influence the quality of a product. It is the totality of the arrangements made with the object of ensuring that pharmaceutical products are of the quality required for their intended use. Quality assurance therefore incorporates GMP and other factors, including those outside the scope of this guide such as product design and development.

The system of quality assurance appropriate to the manufacture of pharmaceutical products should ensure that:

(a) Pharmaceutical products are designed and developed in a way that takes account of the requirements of GMP and other associated codes such as those of good laboratory practice (GLP) and good clinical practice (GCP);

(b) Production and control operations are clearly specified in a written form and GMP requirements are adopted;

(c) Managerial responsibilities are clearly specified in a written form and GMP requirements are adopted.

(d) Arrangements are made for the manufacture, supply and use of the correct starting and packing materials;

(e) All necessary controls on starting materials, intermediate products, and bulk products and other in-process controls, calibrations, and validation are carried out;

(f) The finished product is correctly processed and checked, according to the defined procedures;

(g) Pharmaceutical products are not sold or supplied before the authorized persons have certified that each production batch has been produced and controlled in accordance with the requirements of the marketing authorization and any other regulations relevant to the production, control and release of pharmaceutical products;

(h) Satisfactory arrangements exist to ensure, as far as possible, that the pharmaceutical products are stored by the manufacturer, distributed, and subsequently handled so that quality assurance system;

(i) Deviations are reported, investigated and recorded;

(j) There is a system for approving changes that may have an impact on product quality;

(k) Regular evaluations of the quality of pharmaceutical products should be conducted with the objective of verifying the consistency of the process and ensuring its continuous improvement.

The manufacturer must assume responsibility for the quality of the pharmaceutical products to ensure that they are fit for their intended use, comply with the requirements of the marketing authorization and do not place patients at risk due to inadequate safety, quality or efficacy. The attainment of this quality objective is the responsibility of senior management and requires the participation and commitment of staff in many different departments and at all levels within the company, the company's suppliers, and the distributors. To achieve the quality objective reliably there must be a comprehensively designed and correctly implemented system of a quality assurance incorporating GMP and quality control. It should be fully documented and its effectiveness monitored. All parts of the quality assurance system should be adequately staffed with competent personnel, and should have suitable and sufficient premises, equipment, and facilities.

Quality Control (QC)

The word "Quality" refers to the characteristics of a product from both qualitative and quantitative point of view. It refers to the quality of process as well as the product itself. The word "Control" implies a procedure by which decisions may be made regarding whether production is proceeding according to the plan and meeting the standards established previously. The quality of a pharmaceutical product is a standard, which is designed after a long research and development. Here quality does not concern with active substance alone, but the quality depends upon many other factors such as excipients and product development procedures. The pharmaceutical industry is responsible to design, test and produce dosage form, which provides quality, purity, stability, safety, uniformity of contents and physiological availability to the consumer. Quality control department concerns majorly with the testing and verifying weather the products manufactured (Finished products) and all raw materials, excipients, packaging materials including labels are of quality conforming to the required standards.

The Quality will be checked in the following three different stages

1. Raw material analysis
2. In Process Sample analysis
3. Finished Product analysis

Once the raw material enters the factory premises and before going to the Stores department the Quality of the material will be checked by QC department. If the quality is as per the guidelines, then the QC department approves the raw material. This is called Raw material analysis. The concerned QC chemist will perform the basic duties and the Group leader or Manager approves. The In-Process Analysis will be done while the product (chemical or formulation) is being prepared/ manufactured. Finished product analysis will be done after the product/material is manufactured.

Quality Control is that part of Good Manufacturing Practice which is concerned with sampling, specifications and testing, and with the organisation, documentation and release procedures which ensures that the necessary and relevant tests are actually carried out and that materials are not released for use, nor products released for sale or supply, until their quality has been judged to be satisfactory.

The basic requirements of Quality Control are that:

Adequate facilities, trained personnel and approved procedures are available for sampling and testing starting materials, packaging materials, intermediate, bulk, and finished products, and where appropriate for monitoring environmental conditions for GMP purposes;

Samples of starting materials, packaging materials, intermediate products, bulk products and finished products are taken by approved personnel and methods;

Test methods are validated;

Records are made, manually and/or by recording instruments, which demonstrate that all the required sampling, inspecting and testing procedures were actually carried out. Any deviations are fully recorded and investigated;

The finished products contain active ingredients complying with the qualitative and quantitative composition of the Marketing Authorisation or Clinical Trial Authorisation, are of the purity required, and are enclosed within their proper containers and correctly labelled;

Records are made of the results of inspection and that testing of materials, intermediate, bulk, and finished products is formally assessed against specification. Product assessment includes a review and evaluation of relevant production documentation and an assessment of deviations from specified procedures;

No batch of product is released for sale or supply prior to certification by an Authorised Person that it is in accordance with the requirements of the relevant authorisations;

Sufficient reference samples of starting materials and products are retained in accordance with Annex 19 to permit future examination of the product if necessary and that the sample is retained in the final pack.

Comparison of Quality Assurance and Quality Control

Quality Assurance	Quality Control
QA is a set of activities for ensuring quality in the processes by which products are developed.	QC is a set of activities for ensuring quality in products. The activities focus on identifying defects in the actual products produced.
QA aims to prevent defects with a focus on the process used to make the product. It is a proactive quality process	QC aims to identify (and correct) defects in the finished product. Quality control, therefore, is a reactive process.
The goal of QA is to improve development and test processes so that defects do not arise when the product is being developed	The goal of QC is to identify defects after a product is developed and before it's released.
Establish a good quality management system and the assessment of its adequacy. Periodic conformance audits of the operations of the system	Finding & eliminating sources of quality problems through tools & equipment so that customer's requirements are continually met.
Prevention of quality problems through planned and systematic activities including documentation.	The activities or techniques used to achieve and maintain the product quality, process and service.
Everyone on the team involved in developing the product is responsible for quality assurance	Quality control is usually the responsibility of a specific team that tests the product for defects.

1. Good Manufacturing Practices (GMP) - Principles

Good Manufacturing Practice is that part of Quality Management which ensures that products are consistently produced and controlled to the quality standards appropriate to their intended use and as required by the Marketing Authorisation, Clinical Trial Authorisation or product specification. Good Manufacturing Practice is concerned with both production and quality control.

The basic Requirements (Elements) of GMP are as Follows

(i) All manufacturing processes are clearly defined, systematically reviewed in the light of experience and shown to be capable of consistently manufacturing medicinal products of the required quality and complying with their specifications

(ii) Critical steps of manufacturing processes and significant changes to the process are validated;

(iii) All necessary facilities for GMP are provided including:
- Appropriately qualified and trained personnel
- Adequate premises and space
- Suitable equipment and services
- Correct materials, containers and labels
- Approved procedures and instructions, in accordance with the Pharmaceutical Quality System
- Suitable storage and transport

(iv) Instructions and procedures are written in an instructional form in clear and unambiguous language, specifically applicable to the facilities provided

(v) Procedures are carried out correctly and operators are trained to do so

(vi) Records are made, manually and/or by recording instruments, during manufacture which demonstrate that all the steps required by the defined procedures and instructions were in fact taken and that the quantity and quality of the product was as expected

(vii) Any significant deviations are fully recorded, investigated with the objective of determining the root cause and appropriate corrective and preventive action implemented

(viii) Records of manufacture including distribution which enable the complete history of a batch to be traced are retained in a comprehensible and accessible form

(ix) The distribution of the products minimises any risk to their quality and takes account of good distribution practice

(x) A system is available to recall any batch of product, from sale or supply

(xi) Complaints about products are examined, the causes of quality defects investigated and appropriate measures taken in respect of the defective products and to prevent reoccurrence.

CHPATER - 2

Total Quality Management

Learning Objectives

To learn about

- Definitions of TQM
- Principles and Practices of TQM
- Objectives of TQM
- Elements of TQM
- TQM Philosophy
- Guidelines for Effective TQM Implementation

Definition, Elements and Philosophies

Total quality management (TQM) is a management philosophy that empowers every member of the organization. TQM encourage each individual to participate, contribute and offers to present suggestions for improvement. It is intended to promote continuous and sustained improvement in quality and performance, and develops an attitude of quality culture. Its basic principle is that the cost of prevention is less than the cost of correction. TQM address overall organizational performance and recognizes the importance of processes. For TQM to be successfully adopted by an organization there needs to be a perceived need for change in that organization.

From past few decades, TQM has been extensively discussed in the literature and can be seen as a management philosophy characterized by following principles and practices

(i) Strategies that emphasizes upon continuous improvement in quality,
(ii) Increased involvement of employees,
(iii) Commitment of top management,
(iv) Employee empowerment,
(v) Teamwork,

(vi) Benchmarking,
(vii) Leadership,
(viii) Rewards and recognitions,
(ix) Feedback and relationship with suppliers.

Total Quality Management (TQM) is defined as a participative, systematic management approach to planning and implementing a constant organizational improvement process. Its approach is focused on exceeding customers' expectations, identifying problems, building commitment, and promoting open decision-making among workers.

Total quality management (TQM) is achieved and becomes part of the overall organizational culture when the five principles - produce quality work the first time, focus on the customer, have a strategic approach to improvement, improve continuously and encourage mutual respect and teamwork are implemented.

Total Quality management is defined as a continuous effort by the management as well as employees of a particular organization to ensure long term customer loyalty and customer satisfaction.

Objectives of TQM

TQM integrates the fundamental techniques and principles of quality deployment. The primary objective of TQM is to incorporate quality and integrity into all functions at all levels of the organization.

Elements of TQM

For successful implementation of TQM, an organization must concentrate on the eight key elements namely- Ethics, Integrity, Trust, Training, Teamwork, Leadership, Recognition, Communication.

TQM Philosophy

Total Quality Management (TQM) is a comprehensive system for achieving continuous improvement in customer satisfaction. It is a philosophy of total integration of the business to achieve the required result. The goal is to achieve greater efficiency and effectiveness, lower operating cost and increased market share.

The TQM approach integrates three basic fundamental aspects: commitment, involvement and continuous improvement. Commitment in the sense to take pledge for never ending improvement in quality and services to the customer, involvement means involvement of all the team members in achieving a common goal (i.e. from top to bottom), work as a single unit for better results and think about continuous improvement by looking any error and defects, and eliminating it on spot. TQM addresses the issues of customer satisfaction and guidance on implementing the marketing concept.

TQM is concerned with the integration of all the efforts in the organization towards quality improvement, quality development and quality maintenance to meet full customer satisfaction at all economical levels. TQM enhances quality of work and employer satisfaction through participation and involvement and consequently the image of the organization. It develops participative culture where each employee can directly participate in areas relating to his work and decisions concerning his work. It is organized through quality circles on voluntary basis and quality improvement teams

Guidelines for Effective TQM Implementation

For effective implementation of TQM and better results, following ten basic steps are identified.

(i) Adoption of state-of-art and advanced technologies instead of following traditional culture by the top-management in the organization. Thus, top management commitment is crucial to success.

(ii) Developing quality awareness, imparting training and education on the principles and core concept of TQM to the employees, changing their attitudes and mind set towards quality culture, and commitment of never ending the continuous improvement and innovation in the organization.

(iii) Set the objectives or goals by involving employees at all levels and define them. This will act as the indicators of success in terms of mission.

(iv) Develop and document the approach to TQM and make sure that it is being practiced in the organizations and should not remain on papers only.

(v) Identify the key TQM practices for the organization and create an environment to implement and restrain them by force.

(vi) Prioritize the key TQM practices into different categories and focus on most important practices/categories responsible for improving the organization performance.

(vii) Further, breakdown the key TQM practices into sub-categories, activities, or tasks and form improvement teams.

(viii) Continuously monitor and control the process in response to the difficulties observed from feedback mechanism in the changed process.

(ix) Develop quality improvement teams to solve the quality related issues in quick time without delays. Communicate all the relevant activities, progress and result to the team members and management.

(x) Frequently review and improve the quality plans and measure performance.

CHPATER - 3

ICH Guidelines

Learning Objectives

To learn about

- Purpose and objectives of ICH guidelines
- Participants of ICH Guidelines
- Process of Harmonization
- Brief overview of QSEM guidelines
- ICH Guidelines under Different Series (QSEM)
- Special emphasis on Q series guidelines

Introduction

The International Conference on Harmonization (ICH) is a unique project that brings together the regulatory authorities of Europe, Japan and the United States and experts from the pharmaceutical industry in the three regions to discuss scientific and technical aspects of product registration.

The International Conference on Harmonisation of Technical requirements for the registration of pharmaceuticals for human use (ICH) was established in 1990 as a joint regulatory/industry project to improve, through harmonisation, the efficiency of the process for developing and registering new medicinal products in Europe, Japan and the United States, in order to make these products available to patients with a minimum of delay. The six parties to ICH represent the regulatory bodies and research-based industry in the three regions, Europe, Japan and the USA, where the vast majority of new medicines are currently developed.

The six ICH participants are as follows:

(i) European Commission - European Union (EU).

(ii) European Federation of Pharmaceutical Industries and Associations (EFPIA).

(iii) Ministry of Health, Labour and Welfare, Japan (MHLW).

(iv) Japan Pharmaceutical Manufacturers Association (JPMA).

(v) US Food and Drug Administration (FDA).

(vi) Pharmaceutical Research and Manufacturers of America (PhRMA).

Objectives of ICH Guidelines

- More economical use of human, animal, and material resources.
- Elimination of unnecessary delay in the global development & availability of new medicines.
- Maintaining safeguards on Quality, safety, efficacy and regulatory obligations to protect public health.

Process of Harmonization

- The process of harmonization is a step-wise procedure consisting of the following 5 steps. This procedure is followed for the harmonisation of all new ICH topics.

Step 1: Consensus Building

- The EWG works to prepare a consensus draft of the Technical Document, based on the objectives set out in the Concept Paper. Work is conducted via e-mail, teleconferences and web conferences.
- If endorsed by the ICH Management Committee, the EWG will also meet face-to-face at the time of the biannual Assembly meetings. Interim reports on the progress of the draft are made to the Assembly on a regular basis.

  When consensus on the draft is reached within the EWG, the technical experts of the EWG will sign the *Step 1* Experts sign-off sheet. The *Step 1* Experts Technical Document with EWG signatures is then submitted to the Assembly to request adoption under *Step 2* of the ICH process.

Step 2a: Confirmation of Consensus on the Technical Document

Step 2a is reached when the Assembly agrees, based on the report of the EWG, that there is sufficient scientific consensus on the technical issues for the Technical Document to proceed to the next stage of regulatory consultation.

Step 2b: Adoption of Draft Guideline by Regulatory Members

- On the basis of the Technical Document, the ICH Regulatory Members will take the actions they deem necessary to develop the draft Guideline.
- Step 2b is reached when the Regulatory Members endorse the draft Guideline.

Step 3: Regulatory Consultation and Discussion

- **Step 3 occurs in three distinct stages:** regulatory consultation, discussion and finalisation of the Step 3 Expert Draft Guideline.
- **Stage I - Regional regulatory consultation:** The Guideline embodying the scientific consensus leaves the ICH process and becomes the subject of normal wide-ranging regulatory consultation in the ICH regions. Regulatory authorities and industry associations in other regions may also comment on the draft consultation documents by providing their comments to the ICH Secretariat.
- **Stage II - Discussion of regional consultation comments:** After obtaining all comments from the consultation process, the EWG works to address the comments received and reach consensus on what is called the Step 3 Experts Draft Guideline.
- **Stage III - Finalisation of Step 3 Experts Draft Guideline:** If, after due consideration of the consultation results by the EWG, consensus is reached amongst the experts on a revised version of the Step 2b draft Guideline, the Step 3 Expert Draft Guideline is signed by the experts of the ICH Regulatory Members. The Step 3 Expert Draft Guideline with regulatory EWG signatures is submitted to the Regulatory Members of the Assembly to request adoption as Step 4 of the ICH process.

Step 4: Adoption of an ICH Harmonised Guideline

- Step 4 is reached when the Assembly agrees that there is sufficient consensus on the draft Guideline.
- The Step 4 Final Document is adopted by the ICH Regulatory Members of the ICH Assembly as an ICH Harmonised Guideline at Step 4of the ICH process.

Step 5: Implementation

- Having reached Step 4, the harmonised Guideline moves immediately to the final step of the process that is the regulatory implementation. This step is carried out according to the same national/regional procedures that apply to other regional regulatory guidelines and requirements, in the ICH regions.

Brief Overview of QSEM Guidelines

The ICH guidelines are on the following four categories (QSEM):

(i) Quality (Q series): those relating to chemical and pharmaceutical Quality Assurance (Stability Testing, Impurity Testing, etc.)

(ii) Safety (S series): those relating to in vitro and in vivo pre-clinical studies (Carcinogenicity Testing, Genotoxicity Testing, etc.)

(iii) Efficacy (E series): those relating to clinical studies in human subject (Dose Response Studies, Good Clinical Practices, etc.)

(iv) Multidisciplinary (M series): cross-cutting Topics which do not fit uniquely into one of the above categories (MedDRA, ESTRI, M3, CTD, M5)

The above four categories are summarized in the following table

Q	S	E	M
"Quality" Topics, i.e., those relating to chemical and pharmaceutical quality assurance (Stability Testing, Impurity Testing, etc.)	**"Safety" Topics,** i.e., those relating to in vitro and in vivo pre-clinical studies (Carcinogenicity Testing, Genotoxicity Testing, etc.)	**"Efficacy" Topics,** i.e., those relating to clinical studies in human subject (Dose Response Studies, Good Clinical Practices, etc.)	**"Multidisciplinary" Topics,** i.e., cross cutting Topics which do not fit uniquely into one of the above categories (Med DRA, ESTRI, M3, CTD, M5)

The ICH Guidelines under Different Series are as Follows

1. Quality Guidelines

- Q1A(R2): Stability testing of new drugs and products
- Q1B: Photostability testing
- Q1C: Stability testing of new dosage forms
- Q1D: Bracketing and matrixing designs for stability testing of drug substances and drug products.
- Q1E: Evaluation of stability data
- Q1F: Stability data package for registration in climatic zones III and IV
- Q2A: Definitions and terminology: analytical validation
- Q2B: Methodology

- Q3A(R2): Impurities in new drug substances
- Q3B(R2): Impurities in new drug product
- Q3C(R3): Impurities guidelines for residual solvents
- Q4: Pharmacopoeia
- Q4A: Pharmacopoeial harmonization
- Q5A: Viral safety evaluation
- Q5B: Genetic stability
- Q5C: Stability of biotechnology products
- Q5D: Cell substrates
- Q6A: Specifications, test procedures and acceptance criteria for new drug substances and products
- Q6B: Specification test procedure and acceptance criteria for biotechnological/ biological products
- Q7A: GMP for active pharmaceutical ingredients
- Q8: Pharmaceutical development
- Q9: Quality risk management
- Q10: Pharmaceutical quality system

2. Safety Guidelines

- S1A: Guideline on the need for carcinogenicity studies of pharmaceuticals
- S1B: testing for carcinogenicity of pharmaceuticals
- S1C(R2): Dose selection for carcinogenicity studies of pharmaceuticals
- S2(R1): Guidance on genotoxicity testing and data interpretation for pharmaceuticals intended for human use
- S3A: Note for guidance on toxicokinetics the assessment of systemic exposure in toxicity studies
- S3B: Pharmacokinetics: guidance for repeated dose tissue distribution studies
- S4: Duration of chronic toxicity testing in animals (rodent and nonrodent toxicity testing)
- S5(R2): Detection of toxicity to reproduction for medicinal products & toxicity to male fertility
- S6(R1): Addendum to ICH S6: Preclinical safety evaluation of biotechnology- derived pharmaceuticals

- S6: Preclinical safety evaluation of biotechnology- derived pharmaceuticals
- S7A: Safety pharmacology studies for human pharmaceuticals
- S7B: The non-clinical evaluation of the potential for delayed ventricular repolarization (qt interval prolongation) by human pharmaceuticals
- S8: Immunotoxicity studies for human pharmaceuticals
- S9: Nonclinical evaluation for anticancer pharmaceuticals

3. **Efficacy Guidelines**

- E1: The extent of population exposure to assess clinical safety
- E2A: Clinical safety data management
- E2B(R2): Maintenance of the ich guideline on clinical safety data management
- E2B(R3): Revision of the ich guideline on clinical safety data management
- Data elements for transmission of individual case safety reports
- E2C(R1): Clinical safety data management: periodic safety update reports for marketed drugs
- E2D: Post-approval safety data management: definitions and standards for expedited reporting
- E2E: Pharmacovigilance planning
- E2F: Development safety update report
- E3: Structure and content of clinical study reports
- E4: Dose-response information to support drug registration
- E5(R1): Ethnic factors in the acceptability of foreign clinical data
- E6(R1): Guideline for good clinical practice
- E7: Studies in support of special populations: geriatrics
- E8: General considerations for clinical trials
- E9: Statistical principles for clinical trials
- E10: Choice of control group and related issues in clinical trials
- E11: Clinical investigation of medicinal products in the paediatric population
- E12: Principles for clinical evaluation of new antihypertensive drugs
- E14: The clinical evaluation of qt/qtc interval prolongation and proarrhythmic potential for non-antiarrhythmic drugs

- E15: Definitions for genomic biomarkers, pharmacogenomics, pharmacogenetics, genomic data and sample coding categories
- E16: Genomic biomarkers related to drug response:

4. Multidisciplinary Guidelines

- M1- MedDRA: Medical Terminology
- M2- ESTRI: Electronic Standards for the Transfer of Regulatory Information
- M3- (R2): Nonclinical Safety Studies for the Conduct of Human Clinical Trials and Marketing Authorization for Pharmaceuticals
- M4- CTD: The Common Technical Document
- M5: Data Elements and Standards for Drug Dictionaries

Special Emphasis on Q Series Guidelines

ICH Q series guidelines are those relating to chemical and pharmaceutical Quality Assurance (Stability Testing, Impurity Testing, etc.)

Q1A Q1F are Related to Stability

Q1A: Stability Testing of New Drug Substances and Products

The purpose of stability testing is to provide evidence on how the quality of a drug substance or drug product varies with time under the influence of a variety of environmental factors such as temperature, humidity, and light, and to establish a re-test period for the drug substance or a shelf life for the drug product.

Q1B: Photostability Testing of New Drug Substances and Products

Gives guidance on the basic testing protocol required to evaluate the light sensitivity and stability of new drugs and products

Q1C: Stability Testing for New Dosage Forms

Gives guidelines for new formulations of already approved medicines and defines the circumstances under which reduced stability data can be accepted.

Q1D: Bracketing and Matrixing Designs for Stability Testing of New Drug Substances and Products

Q1E: Evaluation of Stability Data

This guideline addresses the evaluation of stability data that should be submitted in registration applications for new molecular entities and associated drug products. The guideline provides recommendations on establishing shelf lives for drug substances and drug products intended for storage at or below "room temperature".

Q1F: Stability Data Package for Registration Applications in Climatic Zones III and IV

Describes harmonised global stability testing requirements in order to facilitate access to medicines by reducing the number of different storage conditions. WHO conducted a survey amongst their member states to find consensus on 30°C/65% RH as the long-term storage conditions for hot-dry and hot-humid regions.

Q2 are Related to Analytical Validation

Q2(A): Validation of Analytical Procedures: Text and Methodology

The objective of validation of an analytical procedure is to demonstrate that it is suitable for its intended purpose. It Gives validation parameters needed for a variety of analytical methods. It also discusses the characteristics that must be considered during the validation of the analytical procedures. Types of Analytical Procedures to be validated are: Identification tests; Quantitative tests for impurities content; Limit tests for the control of impurities; Quantitative tests of the active moiety in samples of drug substance or drug product or other selected components in the drug product.

Typical validation characteristics of analytical procedures include - Accuracy, Precision (Repeatability, Intermediate Precision), Specificity, Detection Limit, Quantitation Limit, Linearity, Range.

Q3A Q3 are Related to Impurities

Q3A: Impurities in New Drug Substances

The guideline addresses the chemistry and safety aspects of impurities, including the listing of impurities, threshold limit, identification and quantification.

Impurities are of 3 types:

1. Organic impurities (process- and drug-related)
2. Inorganic impurities.
3. Residual solvents

Q3B: Impurities in New Drug Products

Q3C: Impurities Guideline for Residual Solvents

The limit prescribed are as follows:

Benzene 2ppm, Carbon tetrachloride 4ppm, Dichloromethane 5ppm, Dichloroethane 8ppm, Acetonitrile 410ppm, Chloroform 60ppm, Chlorobenzene 360ppm, Toulene 890ppm, Pyridine 200pm, Nitromethane 50ppm, Methanol 3000ppm

Q4 are related to Pharmacopoeias

Q4A: Pharmacopoeial Harmonisation

Q4B: Evaluation and Recommendation of Pharmacopoeial Texts for use in the ICH Regions

This document describes a process for the evaluation and recommendation given by the Q4B Expert Working Group (EWG) for selecting pharmacopoeial texts to facilitate their recognition by regulatory authorities for use, interchangeable in the ICH regions.

Q4B Annex 1: Evaluation and Recommendation of Pharmacopoeial Texts for Use in the ICH Regions on Residue on Ignition/Sulphated Ash

- Annex 2: Test for Extractable Volume of Parenteral Preparations
- Annex 3: Test for Particulate Contamination: Sub-Visible Particles
- Annex 4A: Microbiological Examination of Non-Sterile Products: Microbial Enumeration Tests
- Annex 4B: Microbiological Examination of Non-Sterile Products: Tests for Specified Micro-organisms
- Annex 4C: Microbiological Examination of Non-Sterile Products: Acceptance Criteria for Pharmaceutical Preparations and Substances for Pharmaceutical Use
- Annex 5: Disintegration Test
- Annex 6: Uniformity of Dosage Units
- Annex 7: Dissolution Test
- Annex 8: Sterility Test
- Annex 9: Tablet Friability
- Annex 10: Polyacrylamide Gel Electrophoresis
- Annex 11: Capillary Electrophoresis
- Annex 12: Analytical Sieving
- Annex 13: Bulk Density and Tapped Density of Powders
- Annex14: Bacterial Endotoxins

Q5A Q5E are Related to Quality of Biotechnological Products:

Q5A: Viral Safety Evaluation of Biotechnology Products Derived from Cell Lines of Human or Animal Origin

- This document is concerned with testing and evaluation of the viral safety of biotechnology products derived from cell lines of human or animal origin (i.e., mammalian, avian, insect)

- The objective is to provide a general framework for virus testing experiments for the evaluation ofvirus clearance and the design of viral tests and clearance evaluation studies.
- Three principal, complementary approaches have evolved to control the potential viral contamination of biotechnology products: a) selecting and testing cell lines and other raw materials, including media components, for the absence of undesirable viruses which may be infectious and/or pathogenic for humans; b) Testing the capacity of the processes to clear infectious viruses; c) testing the product at appropriate steps for absence of contaminating infectious viruses.

Q5B: Quality of Biotechnological Products: Analysis of the Expression Construct in Cells used for Production of r-DNA Derived Protein Products

This document presents guidance regarding the characterization of the expression construct for the production of recombinant DNA protein products in eukaryotic and prokaryotic cells. Expression construct should be analyzed using nucleic acid techniques.

Q5C: Quality of Biotechnological Products: Stability Testing of Biotechnological/Biological Products

Q5D: Derivation and Characterization of Cell Substrates used for Production of Biotechnological/Biological Products

- The objective of this guideline is to provide broad guidance on appropriate standards for cell substrates.

Q5E: Comparability of Biotechnological/ Biological Products Subject to Changes in Their Manufacturing Process

- The objective of this document is to provide principles for assessing the comparability of biotechnological/ biological products before and after changes are made in the manufacturing process for the drug substance or drug product.
- Therefore, this guideline is intended to assist in the collection of relevant technical information which serves as evidence that the manufacturing process changes will not have an adverse impact on the quality, safety and efficacy of the drug product.

Q6 are related to Specifications for New Drug Substances and Products

- Bulk drug substance and final product specifications are key parts of the core documentation for world-wide product license applications.

- This leads to conflicting standards for the same product, increased expenses and opportunities for error as well as a potential cause for interruption of product supply.

Q6A: Specifications: Test Procedures and Acceptance Criteria for New Drug Substances and New Drug Products

- The main objective of this guideline is to establish a single set of global specifications for new drug substances and new drug products.
- A specification is defined as a list of tests, references to analytical procedures, and appropriate acceptance criteria, which are numerical limits, ranges
- This guideline addresses specifications, i.e., those tests, procedures, and acceptance criteria which play a major role in assuring the quality of the new drug substance and new drug product during shelf life.

Universal Tests

The following tests are considered generally applicable to all new drug substances and drug products.

- Description
- Identification
- Assay
- Impurities

Specific Tests for Drug Substances

- Physicochemical properties
- Particle size
- Polymorphic forms
- Tests for chiral new drug substances
- Water content
- Inorganic impurities
- Microbial limits

Specific Tests for Drug Products (Oral Dosage Form)

- Particle size distribution
- Dissolution
- Disintegration
- Hardness/friability
- Uniformity of dosage units

- Microbial limits
- Antioxidant preservative content
- Alcohol content Rheological properties Redispersibility
- Specific Tests for drug products (Parenteral Drug Products):
- Uniformity of dosage units
- Particle size distribution
- pH (Osmolarity)
- Sterility
- Endotoxins/Pyrogens
- Particulate matter
- Water content
- Antimicrobial preservative
- Antioxidant preservative content
- Functionality testing of delivery systems

Q6B Specifications: Test Procedures and Acceptance Criteria for Biotechnological/Biological Products

- This document provides guidance on justifying and setting specifications for proteins and polypeptides which are derived from recombinant or non-recombinant cell cultures.
- A valid biological assay to measure the biological activity should be provided by the manufacturer.
- Examples of procedures used to measure biological activity include:
- Animal-based biological assays, which measure an organism's biological response to the product;
- Cell culture-based biological assays, which measure biochemical or physiological response at the cellular level;
- Biochemical assays, which measure biological activities such as enzymatic reaction rates or biological responses induced by immunological interactions.

Q7 are related to Good Manufacturing Practice Guide for Active Pharmaceutical Ingredients

The main objective of this guideline is that to maintain the quality of the:

- Active pharmaceutical ingredients
- Personnel
- Buildings and Facilities
- Process equipment
- Documentation and Records

Q8 are related to Pharmaceutical Development

This guideline is intended to provide guidance on the contents of Pharmaceutical Development of drug products. The aim of pharmaceutical development is to design a quality product and its manufacturing process to consistently deliver the intended performance of the product. The Pharmaceutical Development section also describes the type of dosage form and the formulation that are suitable for the intended use. Q8 gives information about Drug Substance, Excipients, and Container Closure System.

Q9 are Related to Quality Risk Management

The purpose of this document is to offer a systematic approach to quality risk management. This guideline provides principles and tools for quality risk management that can be applied to all aspects of pharmaceutical quality including development, manufacturing, distribution; and the inspection and submission/review processes throughout the lifecycle of drug substances and drug (medicinal) products, biological and biotechnological products, including the use of raw materials, solvents, excipients, packaging and labelling materials.

Q10 are Related to Pharmaceutical Quality System

This document establishes a new ICH tripartite guideline describing a model for an effective quality management system for the pharmaceutical industry, referred to as the Pharmaceutical Quality System.

Comprehensive model for an effective pharmaceutical quality system is based on International Standards Organization (ISO) quality concepts, includes applicable Good Manufacturing Practice (GMP) regulations.

CHPATER - 4

ICH Stability Testing Guidelines and Procedures

Learning Objectives

To learn about

- Stability and Stability testing of Pharmaceuticals
- Importance of Stability Testing
- Stability Testing Methods
- Real Time Stability Testing
- Accelerated Stability Testing
- Retained Sample Stability Testing
- Climatic Zones for Stability Testing
- Protocol for Stability Testing
- Sampling Plan
- Test Storage conditions
- Test Parameters
- Test Methodology
- Conduct of Stability Studies
- Photo Stability Testing
- Stability Test Equipment

Stability testing of pharmaceutical products is a complex set of procedures involving considerable cost, time consumption and scientific expertise in order to build in quality, efficacy and safety in a drug formulation. The most important step during the developmental stages include stability studies that are required to determine and assure the identity, potency and purity of ingredients, as well as those of the formulated products. Stability of a pharmaceutical product may be defined as the capability of a particular formulation in a specific container/closure system to remain within its physical, chemical, microbiological, toxicological, protective and informational specifications. In other words, it is the extent to which a product retains, within the specified limits, throughout its period of storage and use, the same properties and characteristics possessed at the time of its packaging. Stability testing thus evaluates the effect of environmental factors on the quality of the a drug substance or a formulated product which is utilized for prediction of its shelf life, determine proper storage conditions and suggest labeling instructions. Moreover, the data generated during the stability testing is an important requirement for regulatory approval of any drug or formulation.

Importance of Stability Testing

The primary reason for stability testing is the concern for the well-being of the patient suffering from the disease for which the products is designed. Apart from degradation of the unstable product into toxic decomposition products, loss of activity up to a level of 85% of that claimed on the label may lead to failure of the therapy resulting in death e.g. nitroglycerine tablets for angina and cardiac arrest. Because of this concern, it has become a legal requirement to provide data for certain types of stability tests for the regulatory agencies before approval of a new product. Second important concern is to protect the reputation of the manufacturer by assuring that the product will retain fitness for use with respect to all functionally relevant attributes for as long as they are on the market. Other benefits of stability studies at the developmental stage or of the marketed products are to provide a database that may be of value in selection of adequate formulations, excipients and container closure systems for development of a new product, to determine shelf life and storage conditions for development of a new product, preparation of registration dossier, to substantiate the claimed shelf life for the registration dossier and to verify that no changes have been introduced in the formulation or manufacturing process that can adversely affect the stability of the product .

Stability Testing Methods

Stability testing is a routine procedure performed on drug substances and products and is employed at various stages of the product development. In early stages, accelerated stability testing (at relatively high temperatures and/or humidity) is used in order to determine the type of degradation products which may be found after long-term storage. Testing under less rigorous conditions i.e. those recommended for long-term shelf storage, at slightly elevated temperatures is used to determine a product's shelf life and expiration dates. The major aim of pharmaceutical stability testing is to provide reasonable assurance that the products will remain at an acceptable level of fitness/quality throughout the period during which they are in market place available for supply to the patients and will be fit for their consumption until the patient uses the last unit of the product. Depending upon the aim and steps followed, stability testing procedures have been categorized into the following four types.

Real-Time Stability Testing

Real-time stability testing is normally performed for longer duration of the test period in order to allow significant product degradation under recommended storage conditions. The period of the test depends upon the stability of the product which should be long enough to indicate clearly that no measurable degradation occurs and must permit one to distinguish degradation from inter-assay variation. During the testing, data is collected at an appropriate frequency such that a trend analysis is able to distinguish instability from day-to-day ambiguity. The reliability of data interpretation can be increased by including a single batch of reference material for which stability characteristics have already been established. Stability of the reference material also includes the stability of reagents as well as consistency of the performance of the instrument to be used throughout the period of stability testing. However, system performance and control for drift and discontinuity resulting from changes in both reagents and instrumentation must be monitored.

Accelerated Stability Testing

In accelerated stability testing, a product is stressed at several high (warmer than ambient) temperatures and the amount of heat input required to cause product failure is determined. This is done to subject the product to a condition that accelerates degradation. This information is then projected to predict shelf life or used to compare the relative stability of alternative formulations. This usually provides an early indication of the product shelf life and thus shortening the development schedule. In addition to temperature, stress conditions applied during accelerated stability testing are moisture, light, agitation, gravity, pH and package. In accelerated stability testing the samples are subjected to stress, refrigerated after stressing, and then assayed simultaneously. Because the duration of the analysis is short, the likelihood of instability in the measurement system is reduced in comparison to the real-time stability testing. Further, in accelerated stability testing, comparison of the unstressed product with stressed material is made within the same assay and the stressed sample recovery is expressed as percent of unstressed sample recovery. For statistical reasons, the treatment in accelerated stability projections is recommended to be conducted at four different stress temperatures. However, for thermolabile and proteinaceous components, relatively accurate stability projections are obtained when denaturing stress temperatures are avoided.

The concept of accelerated stability testing is based upon the Arrhenius equation (1) and modified Arrhenius equation (2):

$$\ln A + \frac{\Delta E}{RT}$$

$$\ln K = A + \frac{\Delta E}{RT} \qquad .....(4.1)$$

where K = degradation rate/s, A = frequency factor/s, ΔE = activation energy (kJ/mol), R = universal gas constant (0.00831 kJ/mol), T= absolute temperature (K)

$$\log\left(\frac{K_2}{K_1}\right)\left(\frac{1}{T_2} \quad \frac{1}{T_1}\right) \qquad .....(4.2)$$

$$-E_a = 2303R$$

where *k1* and *k2* are rate constants at temperatures *T1* and *T2* expressed in degree kelvins; Ea is the activation energy; R is the gas constant.

These equations describe the relationship between storage temperatures and degradation rate. Using Arrhenius equation, projection of stability from the degradation rates observed at high temperatures for some degradation processes can be determined. When the activation energy is known, the degradation rate at low temperatures may be projected from those observed at "stress" temperatures. The stress tests used in the current International Conference on Harmonization (ICH) guideline (e.g., 40% for products to be stored at controlled room temperature) were developed from a model that assumes energy of activation of about 83 kJ per mole.

Retained Sample Stability Testing

This is a usual practice for every marketed product for which stability data are required. In this study, stability samples, for retained storage for at least one batch a year are selected. If the number of batches marketed exceeds 50, stability samples from two batches are recommended to be taken. At the time of first introduction of the product in the market, the stability samples of every batch may be taken, which may be decreased to only 2% to 5% of marketed batches at a later stage. In this study, the stability samples are tested at predetermined intervals i.e. if a product has shelf life of 5 years, it is conventional to test samples at 3, 6, 9, 12,18, 24, 36, 48, and 60 months. This conventional method of obtaining stability data on retained storage samples is known as constant interval method. Stability testing by evaluation of market samples is a modified method which involves taking samples already in the market place and evaluating stability attributes. This type of testing is inherently more realistic since it challenges the product not just in the idealized retained sample storage conditions, but also in the actual marketplace.

Cyclic Temperature Stress Testing

This is not a routine testing method for marketed products. In this method, cyclic temperature stress tests are designed on knowledge of the product so as to mimic likely conditions in market place storage. The period of cycle mostly considered is 24 hours since the diurnal rhythm on earth is 24 hour, which the marketed pharmaceuticals are most likely to experience during storage. The minimum and maximum temperatures for the cyclic stress testing is recommended to be selected on a product- by-product basis and considering factors like recommended storage temperatures for the product and specific chemical and physical degradation properties of the products. It is also recommended that the test should normally have 20 cycles.

Climatic Zones for Stability Testing

For the purpose of stability testing, the whole world has been divided into four zones (I - IV) depending upon the environmental conditions the pharmaceutical products are likely to be subjected to during their storage. These conditions have been derived on the basis of the mean annual temperature and relative humidity data in these regions. Based upon this data, long-term or real-time stability testing conditions and accelerated stability testing conditions have been derived. The standard climatic zones for use in pharmaceutical product stability studies have been presented in the Table 4.

Protocol for Stability Testing

The protocol for stability testing is a pre-requisite for starting stability testing and is necessarily a written document that describes the key components of a regulated and well-controlled stability study. Because the testing condition is based on inherent stability of the compound, the type of dosage form and the proposed container-closure system, the protocol depends on the type of drug substance or the product. In addition, the protocol can depend on whether the drug is new or is already in the market. The protocol should also reflect the regions where the product is proposed to be marketed e.g. if the product is planned to be used in climatic zones I-III, IVa and IVb, the stability program must include all these zones. A well designed stability protocol should contain the following information.

Batches

Stability studies at developmental stages are generally carried out on a single batch while studies intended for registration of new product or unstable established product are done on first three production batches, while for stable and well-established batches, even two are allowed. If the initial data is not on a full- scale production batch, first three batches of drug product manufactured post-approval should be placed on long-term studies using the same protocol as in approved drug application. Data on laboratory scale batches obtained during development of pharmaceuticals are not accepted as primary stability data but constitute supportive information. In general, the selection of batches should constitute a random sample from the population of pilot or production batches.

Containers and Closures

The testing is done on the product in immediate containers and closures proposed for marketing. The packaging materials include aluminium strip packs, blister packs, Alu-Alu packs, HDPE bottles etc. This may also include secondary packs, but not shippers. Products in all different types of containers/closures, whether meant for distribution or for physician and promotional samples, are to be tested separately. However, for bulk containers, testing in prototype containers is allowed, if it simulates the actual packaging.

Orientation of Storage of Containers

Samples of the solutions, dispersed systems and semi solid drug products for stability studies must be kept upright and positioned either inverted or on the side to allow for full interaction of the product with the container-closure. This orientation helps to determine whether the contact between the drug product or solvent and the closure results in the extraction of chemical substances from the closure components or adsorption of product components into the container-closure.

Sampling Time Points

Frequency of testing should be such that it is sufficient to establish the stability profile of the new drug substance. For products with a proposed shelf life of at least 12 months, the testing frequency at the long-term storage condition should be every 3 months over the first year, every 6 months over the second year and annually thereafter throughout the proposed shelf life expiration date. In the case of accelerated storage conditions, a minimum of three time points, including the initial and end points, for example, 0, 3, and 6 months is recommended. When testing at the intermediate storage condition is necessary as a result of significant change at the accelerated storage condition, a minimum of four test points, including the initial and final time points, is recommended, for example, 0, 6, 9 and 12 months. The test schedule for stability testing of a new product has been presented in Table 5.

In case the same product of different strengths, multiple sizes, etc is required to be tested, reduced stability testing plans can be worked out, which involves less number of test points. The reduced testing plans are based on bracketing and matrixing statistical designs. Bracketing is the design of a stability schedule such that only samples on the extremes of certain design factors, e.g., strength, package size, are tested at all time points as in a full design. On the other hand, matrixing involves testing of a subset of the total number of possible samples for all combinations at a specific time point. Subsequently, another subset of samples for all factor combinations is tested. The factors that can be matrixed include batches, strengths with identical formulation, container sizes, fill sizes, and intermediate time points.

Sampling Plan

Sampling plan for stability testing involves, planning for the number of samples to be charged to the stability chambers and sampling out of the charged batch so as to cover the entire study. The first step should be the development of the sampling time points followed by the number of samples needed to be drawn at each pull point for complete evaluation of all test parameters and finally adding up to get the total number of samples. For example there would be a requirement of about 100 tablets per pull out in a long term or accelerated stability studies including 10 each for assay, hardness and moisture determination, 6 each for dissolution and disintegration and 50 for friability. This multiplied by the total number of pull outs will give the total number of tablets required for a study. This is followed by the development of a sampling plan, which includes the selection of the containers representing the batch as a whole but in an unbiased manner. A stratification plan has been suggested whereby from a random starting point every nth container is taken from the filling or packaging line (n is chosen such that the sample is spread over the whole batch).

Test Storage Conditions

The storage conditions to be selected are based upon the climatic zone in which the product is intended to be marketed or for which the product is proposed to be filed for regulatory approval. General recommendations on the storage conditions have been given by ICH, CPMP and WHO. The abridged/indicative ICH and WHO storage conditions for drug products have been given in

Test Parameters

The stability test protocol should define the test parameters that would be used for evaluation of the stability samples. The tests that monitor the quality, purity, potency, and identity which could be expected to change upon storage are chosen as stability tests. Therefore appearance, assay, degradation products, microbiological testing, dissolution, and moisture are standard tests performed on stability test samples. Microbiological tests include sterility, preservative efficacy and microbial count as applicable e.g. for liquid injectable preparations. The batches used for stability study must meet all the testing requirements including heavy metals, residue on ignition, residual solvents etc. Some of these are required at the time of product release but not required to be repeated during stability testing. Other tests like enantiomeric purity, particle size and polymorphic form etc have also been discussed in ICH guidance Q6A.

Test Methodology

It is always recommended to follow the procedures given in the official compendia, as the results obtained using the official tests, in general find better acceptance. If alternate methods are used, they are required to be duly validated. However, the assay of the drug should be carried out using a stability-indicating method, established by carrying out stress tests on the drug under forced decomposition conditions. The methods reported in literature should be used after confirming reproducibility and carrying out minimal validation, say of linearity, range, etc. It is always recommended to prepare a standard test protocol (STP) for each test.

Acceptance Criteria

All analytical methods are required to be validated before initiating the stability studies. Similarly, the acceptance criteria for the analytical results as well as that for the presence of degradation products should also be fixed beforehand. The acceptance criteria for each test in the stability study is fixed in the form of numerical limits for the results expressed in quantitative terms e.g., moisture pick-up, viscosity, particle size, assay, degradation products, etc. and pass or fail for qualitative tests e.g., odour, colour, appearance, cracking, microbial growth, etc. These acceptance criteria should also include individual and total upper limits for degradation products. ICH guideline Q3B (R2) related to impurities in new drug products addresses degradation products in new drug formulations. The degradation products of the active or interaction products from the active ingredients and excipients and/or active and container component should be reported, identified, and/or qualified when the proposed thresholds are exceeded. The reporting threshold of impurities is based upon the intended dose. If the maximum daily dose is less than or equal to 1gm, the limit is 0.1% and if greater than 1, the limit is 0.05%. The identification threshold of impurities is between 1.0-0.1% for the maximum daily dose ranging between 1mg and 2mg.

Conduct of Stability Studies

The stability study is conducted by keeping the drug substance or the product in their proposed final packs (e.g. Aluminium strip, blister pack, Alu-Alu pack, HDPE container etc.), or prototype containers in the case of bulk drugs, in sufficient numbers in the stability chambers set at appropriate storage conditions as per the protocol. The samples are then withdrawn, as per the stability protocol, at the prescribed sampling intervals and are then analyzed by a suitable method. The sampling should preferably be from unopened container. As far as possible the samples are placed for testing as soon as they have been prepared and analyzed without delay after they have been withdrawn. Delay in placing the samples and analysis of withdrawn samples is known to affect the results. However, if there is an unavoidable delay, then the samples are frozen until they are subjected to analysis. In order to minimize the effect of day-to-day variability on the results, the following two approaches are followed. Samples are drawn in replicate. One of the samples is tested and others are kept at temperatures sufficiently low to prevent further drug loss and then all the samples are subjected to analysis on the same day at the end of study (i.e. after withdrawal of the last sample).

Second approach is to freeze the initial samples till the expiration period and test them at appropriate times by using them as internal standards in the assays.

Photo Stability Testing

USA FDA in 1996 issued ICH guidance for industry and stated that "the intrinsic photostability characteristics of new drug substances and products should be evaluated to demonstrate that, as appropriate, light exposure does not result in unacceptable change". In this photostability testing is recommended to be carried out on a single batch of material, however these studies should be repeated if certain variations and changes are made to the product (e.g., formulation, packaging). While D65 is the internationally recognized standard for outdoor daylight as defined in ISO 10977 (1993), ID65 is the equivalent indoor indirect daylight standard. Following this, testing of drugs in photostability chamber is now increasingly being followed as a standard procedure, especially for the products intended to be marketed in Asian countries.

Stability Test Equipment

The equipment used for stability testing is called stability chamber. These are specialized environmental chambers that can simulate the storage condition and enable evaluation of product stability based on real-time, accelerated and long-term protocols. They are available in both walk-in and reach-in styles. Smaller chambers are preferred for accelerated testing, as the retention time of products is much less in these cabinets, while the walk-in chambers are preferred for long-term testing. Such chambers or rooms are engineered and qualified to ensure uniform exposure of the set conditions to all the samples in the chamber. These chambers are expected to be dependable and rugged because of the requirement of uninterrupted use for years. They are fitted with appropriate recording, safety and alarm devices. In addition, photostability chambers are also available and utilized both with and without temperature and humidity control. Two types of light sources are usually employed in photostability chambers, one is the combination of cool white and near UV fluorescent tubes, while second are the artificial daylight lamps, e.g., xenon or metal halide. It is required to obtain a total exposure of 1.2 million lux hours. The visible light intensity is estimated using a lux meter. The calculation is made on how many hours of exposure is needed.

CHPATER - 5

Quality by Design (QbD)

Learning Objectives

To learn about

- Definition and concept of QbD
- Implementation of QbD
- Elements of QbD
- Critical Quality Attributes
- Design Space
- Critical process parameters
- Tools of QbD
- Risk Assesment
- Design of Experiment (DOE)
- Process Analytical Technology (PAT)
- Key charecteristics of QbD
- Benefits of QbD

Quality by Design (QbD) is increasingly becoming an important and widely used technique in the pharmaceutical industry. QbD can be considered to be systems-based approach to the design, development, and delivery of any product or service to a consumer. QbD is a systematic approach to pharmaceutical development that begins with predefined objectives and emphases product and process understanding and process control. It means designing and developing formulations and manufacturing processes to ensure predefined product quality objectives. QbD identifies characteristics that are critical to quality from the perspective of patients, translates them into the attributes that the drug product should possess and establish how the critical process parameters can be varied to consistently produce a drug product with the desired characteristics. The main concept of QbD is that all final product-critical quality attributes are affected by raw materials and process parameters. Hence, if we identify the cause and effect relationship between various inputs and the responses by carefully designed experiments, we can control the quality of the product by simply controlling the inputs like raw material specifications or process parameters etc. As a result, the final product will always conform to the quality specifications.

Quality by Design Implementation

The first step in implementing Quality by Design system is understanding the cause and effect relationship between the raw material attributes, process conditions and the critical quality attributes of the final product by employing design of experiments (DOE). There are several designs of experiments that are available in any commercial software that a formulator can use. Examples- factorial designs, Taguchi designs, mixture designs, response surface designs, etc. And within each design there several options available for the formulator to suit the needs and goals of the experiments. Examples: Blocking, confounding, fractional factorial, 3 factorials, Placket-Burmann designs, Latin Squares design, etc

After the designed experiments are executed, the results are analyzed and studied to identify the cause and effect relationships between input parameters and responses. The next step in implementing QbD is scaling up the experiments either to the manufacturing level or intermediate level. In this processes, one can use prior knowledge to run fractional designs that will eliminate the need to run several large-scale experiments.

The last step in implementation of QbD is defining the control strategies for raw materials and manufacturing process parameters. The implementation of control strategy inherently addresses the implementation of design space. If certain inputs, such as excipient particle size or drug crystal surface area, are related to the performance of the final product, then it is logical, in QbD, to control the particle size or surface area to the ranges dictated by the experiments. Once the control strategies are identified, manufacturer should procure, install, commission and validate the control systems to implement QbD.

Elements of Quality by Design

Various elements of quality by design as described in ICH Q8 (R2) include Target product profile, Identification of quality attributes, Risk assessment to identify process/product risk, Design space development and Control strategies.

Identifying a Quality Target Product Profile (QTPP)

The quality target product profile (QTPP) is a summary of the quality characteristics or attributes of a drug product that ideally will be achieved and thereby ensure the safety and efficacy of a drug product. The QTPP forms the basis of design for the development of the product. It is both prospective, that is, it describes the goals for the development team, and dynamic, that is, the QTPP may be updated or revised at various stages of development as new information is obtained during the development process.

Identification of Critical Quality Attributes (CQA)

Pharmaceutical development consists of product and process design and development. The TPP provides the basis for the ideal dosage form. A critical quality attribute is a physical, chemical, biological, or microbiological property or characteristic that should be within an appropriate limit, range, or distribution to ensure the desired product quality. CQAs are generally associated with raw materials (drug substance, excipients), intermediates (in-process materials), and drug product. Drug product CQAs are the properties that are important for product performance, that is, the desired quality, safety, and efficacy.

Quality Attributes Important to the Performance of the Drug Product

From a clinical perspective, safety and efficacy (product performance) is of prime importance. For example for an oral CR product, it is important to consider attributes that are potentially critical for performance. These may be drug dissolution/release, potency, polymer concentration, polymer viscosity, glass transition temperature (Tg) of composite, etc., or any other attribute that can either be substituted for drug release or clinical performance.

Quality Risk Assessment

A key objective of risk assessment in pharmaceutical development is to identify which material attributes and process parameters affect the drug product CQAs, that is, to understand and predict sources of variability in the manufacturing process so that an appropriate control strategy can be implemented to ensure that the CQAs are within the desired requirements.

Critical Process Parameters

A critical process parameter (CPP) is any measurable input (input material attribute or operating parameter) or output (process state variable or output material attribute) of a process step that must be controlled to achieve the desired product quality and process consistency.

For example the following are the process parameters and material attributes related to wet granulation process:

1. Attributes related drug substance: Amount, Form, Particle size, Moisture content and Bulk density.
2. Attributes related to excipients: Excipient amount, Excipient particle size and Excipient density.
3. Granulation operating parameters: Chopper configuration, Impellor speed, Granulation time, Temperature, Spray nozzle type and Binder addition rate.
4. Granulation state conditions: Power consumption and Temperature.
5. Attributes after granulation: Blend uniformity, Granule size distribution, Agglomerate size, Moisture, Bulk density and Flow properties.

A parameter is critical when a realistic change in that parameter can cause the product to fail to meet the TPQP. Thus, whether a parameter is critical or not depends on how large of a change one is willing to consider. Thus, the first step in classifying parameters is to define the range of interest which we call the potential operating space (POS). The POS is the region between the maximum and minimum value of interest for each process parameter. Criteria for identifying critical and non-critical parameters are that a parameter is non-critical when there is no trend to failure within the POS and there is no evidence of interactions within the proven acceptable range (PAR), which is the range of experimental observations that lead to acceptable quality.

Design Space

Design Space is defined as the multidimensional combination of input variables (e.g., material attributes) and process parameters that have been demonstrated to provide assurance of quality. Working within the design space is not considered as a change. Movement out of the design space is considered to be a change and would normally initiate a regulatory post approval change process. Design space is proposed by the applicant and is subject to regulatory assessment and approval.

Control Strategy

A control strategy normally include input material controls, process controls and monitoring, design space around individual or multiple unit operations, and/or final product specifications used to ensure consistent quality. The finished drug products are tested for quality by assessing if they meet specifications. In addition, manufacturers are usually expected to conduct extensive in process tests, such as blend uniformity or tablet hardness.

Tools of QbD

The concept of QbD has two components – the science underlying the design and the science of manufacturing. Upon understanding the elements of QbD and the steps for QbD implementation, it is important to be familiar with the commonly used tools in QbD, including risk assessment, design of experiment (DoE), and process analytical technology (PAT).

Risk Assessment

Risk assessment is a systematic process of organizing information to support a risk decision to be made within a risk asessment, either separately or in combination. The risk factors in the fishbone diagram are classified into broad categories, while the FMEA could identify the failure modes that have the greatest chance of causing product failure, which means each of the factors in the Ishikawa fishbone diagrams will be ranked later in the FMEA analysis. The FMEA method can be used to perform the quantitative risk assessment, identifying the CQAs that have the greatest chance of causing product failure. The outcome of an FMEA are risk priority numbers (RPN) for each combination of failure mode severity, occurrence probability, and likelihood of detection.

Design of Experiment (DoE)

To carry out the design of experiment, the risk assessment should be taken into function first. A structured, organized method for determining the relationship between factors affecting a process and the output of that process is known as "Design of Experiments" (DoE). DoE is an excellent tool that allows pharmaceutical scientists to systematically manipulate factors according to a pre-specified design. A good design is based on sound cognition of product and effective management of whole process during manufacturing. DoE studies work together with mechanism-based studies to achieve better product and process understanding.

DoE is a reasonable method to determine the relationship between the inputs and outputs of a process. It can help identify optimal conditions, CMAs, CPPs, and, ultimately, the Design Space. It is wise to establish a Design Space through DoE for multivariate experiments. ICH Q8 defines the Design Space as "the multidimensional combination and interaction of input variables (e.g., material attributes) and process parameters that have been demonstrated to provide assurance of quality". It has been reported that there is no need to hand over supplements to revise (e.g., widen) the acceptance criteria to FDA if the changes are within the Design Space.

So far, a number of studies have been launched in the drug delivery systems after QbD initiative was claimed. It has been demonstrated that DoE is effective in the design of different dosage forms and unit operations, it can be used more broadly in the near future to guarantee high research efficiency with improved product quality.

PAT as an Important Tool of QbD

PAT is defined as "Tools and systems that utilize real-time measurements, or rapid measurements during processing, of evolving quality and performance attributes of in-process materials to provide information to ensure optimal processing to produce final product that consistently conforms to established quality and performance standards". ICH Q8 identifies the use of PAT to ensure that the process remains within an established Design Space.

The concept originates from the desire of the regulators to shift control of product quality toward a science-based approach that explicitly attempts to reduce the risk to patients by controlling the manufacturing based on understanding of the process.

From a PAT standpoint, a process is considered well understood when

1. All critical sources of variability are identified and explained;
2. Variability is managed by the process; and
3. Product quality attributes can be accurately and reliably predicted.

PAT Steps

There is a three-step-process in the design and optimization of drug formulations and manufacturing processes, namely design, analyze and control.

In the design step, experimentation is performed to under- stand which quality attributes are related to a given unit operation and which process parameters and raw material attributes have the most impact on the final product quality. This knowledge is then used to identify the QTPP, CPP and CQA, which are needed for consideration in the design of an effective PAT based control scheme for the process.

In the analysis step, to identify the chosen quality attribute and process parameters and the raw material attributes, a process measurement system allows for real time (or near real time) monitoring of all CQAs and CPPs, using direct or in-direct analytical methods with appropriate analytical tools.

Finally, control strategies provide adjustments to ensure control of all critical attributes, and set up the understanding of relationships among CQAs, CPPs and QTPPs so as to decide what action to take in case the process performance deviates from the optimal path or product quality from the desired attributes.

PAT Tools

For the sake of understanding scientific, risk-managed pharmaceutical development, manufacture and quality assurance, many tools are available in the PAT framework. They can be categorized into four classes according to the PAT guidance:

1. Multivariate tools for design, data acquisition and analysis;
2. Process analyzers;
3. Process control tools;
4. Continuous improvement and knowledge management tools.

As defined by FDA's PAT guidance document, whether to remove the sample or not, process analysis can be divided into three categories, namely at-line, on-line and in-line: (1) At-line: Measurement where the sample is removed, isolated from, and analyzed in close proximity to the process stream; (2) On- line: Measurement where the sample is diverted from the manufacturing process, and may be returned to the process stream; (3) In-line: Measurement where the sample is not removed from the process stream and can be invasive or noninvasive.

It is obvious that PAT is definitely effective in helping QbD implement. It can do a job of real time monitoring of process without interruption to get technological parameters and material parameters online. PAT enhances understanding of technology (including the relationship between CQA and CPP), which leads to accomplishment of quality improvement and register simplification.

Application of PAT

In most cases, spectroscopic techniques, including Raman spectroscopy, UV–VIS spectroscopy, and nuclear magnetic resonance (NMR), are commonly used. Besides, other PAT analytical methods, such as Near Infrared spectroscopy (NIR), focused beam reflectance measurements (FBRM), nanometric temperature measurement (NTM), tunable diode laser absorption spectroscopy (TDLAS), are widely applied in the pharmaceutical manufacturing field and play important roles in the real-time monitoring of the processes. Among those PAT tools, NIR has drawn great attention in the pharmaceutical industry, it is a rapid, non-invasive analytical technique and there is no need for extensive sample preparation. NIR has been described in both the United States and the European

Pharmacopeia. It is the most commonly used device in the manufacturing process, and it has been used for the identification and characterization of raw materials and intermediates, analysis of dosage forms manufacturing, and prediction of one or more variables in process streams or final product streams (composition) on the basis of on-line, in-line or at-line spectroscopic measurements. Due to the complexity of pharmaceutical product-process design, an efficient and systematic understanding coupled with an inference system is essential. The real-time monitoring tools have increasingly attracted the interests of pharmaceutical manufacturers. So far, the continuous manufacturing and real-time monitoring are mostly used in the tablet manufacturing processes.

Key Characteristics of QbD

- A tool for focused & efficient drug development
- Dynamic and systematic process
- Relies on the concept that Quality can be built in as a continuum
- It is applicable to Drug Product and Drug Substance development (chemicals / biologics)
- It is applicable to analytical methods
- Can be implemented partially or totally
- Can be used at any time in the life cycle of the Drug
- Always encouraged by Regulators.

Benefits of QbD

- Eliminate batch failures
- Minimize deviations and costly investigations
- Avoid regulatory compliance problems
- Empowerment of technical staff
- Efficient, agile, flexible system
- Increase manufacturing efficiency, reduce costs and project rejections and waste
- Build scientific knowledge base for all products
- Better interact with industry on science issues
- Ensure consistent information
- Incorporate risk management
- Reduce end-product testing
- Speed-up release decision

CHPATER - 6

ISO 9000 and ISO 14000

Learning Objectives

To learn about:

- ISO- Overview
- ISO 9000 – ISO 9001
- Quality Management Principles
- ISO 14000- ISO 14001
- Environmental Management
- ISO Certification and Registration
- ISO Accreditation
- Benefits of ISO 9001 and 14001
- ISO Registration Process (Steps for Registration)
- ISO Auditors
- NABL Accreditation – Principles and Benefits
- Procedures (Steps to Accreditation)

ISO - Overview

ISO (International Organization for Standardization) is a worldwide federation of national standards bodies. ISO is a nongovernmental organization that comprises standards bodies from more than 160 countries, with one standards body representing each member country. The American National Standards Institute (ANSI) for example, represents the United States. Member organizations collaborate in the development and promotion of international standards for technology, scientific testing processes, working conditions, societal issues and more. ISO and its members then sell documents detailing these standards. A General Assembly, which consists of representatives from ISO members and elected leaders called principal officers, acts as the decision-making body for ISO. The organization has its headquarters in Geneva, Switzerland, where a central secretariat oversees operations.

ISO 9001 and ISO 14001 are among ISO's most well-known standards ever. They are implemented by more than a million organizations in some 175 countries. ISO 9001 helps organizations to implement quality management.ISO 14001 helps organizations to implement environmental management.

The ISO 9000 series are based on seven quality management principles. The seven quality management principles are:

QMP 1 – Customer focus

QMP 2 – Leadership

QMP 3 – Engagement of people

QMP 4 – Process approach

QMP 5 – Improvement

QMP 6 – Evidence-based decision making

QMP 7 – Relationship management

Principle 1 – Customer focus Organizations depend on their customers and therefore should understand current and future customer needs, should meet customer requirements and strive to exceed customer expectations.

Principle 2 – Leadership - Leaders establish unity of purpose and direction of the organization. They should create and maintain the internal environment in which people can become fully involved in achieving the organization's objectives.

Principle 3 – Engagement of people - People at all levels are the essence of an organization and their full involvement enables their abilities to be used for the organization's benefit.

Principle 4 – Process approach - A desired result is achieved more efficiently when activities and related resources are managed as a process

Principle 5 – Improvement - Improvement of the organization's overall performance should be a permanent objective of the organization.

Principle 6 – Evidence-based decision making Effective decisions are based on the analysis of data and information.

Principle 7 – Relationship management An organization and its external providers (suppliers, contractors, service providers) are interdependent and a mutually beneficial relationship enhances the ability of both to create value.

Quality Management

ISO 9001 is for quality management. Quality refers to all those features of a product (or service) which are required by the customer. Quality management means what the organization does to ensure that its products or services satisfy the customer's quality requirements and comply with any regulations applicable to those products or services. Quality management also means what the organization does to enhance customer satisfaction and achieve continual improvement of its performance.

Environmental Management

ISO 14001 is for environmental management. This means what the organization does to minimize harmful effects on the environment caused by its activities, to conform to applicable regulatory requirements, and to achieve continual improvement of its environmental performance.

Generic Standards

ISO 9001 and ISO 14001 are generic standards. Generic means that the same standards can be applied: to any organization, large or small, whatever its product or service, in any sector of activity, and whether it is a business enterprise, a public administration, or a government department. Generic also signifies that no matter what the organization's scope of activity if it wants to establish a quality management system, ISO 9001 gives the essential features or if it wants to establish an environmental management system, ISO 14001 gives the essential features.

Management Systems

Management system means what the organization does to manage its processes, or activities in order that its products or services meet the organization's objectives, such as satisfying the customer's quality requirements, complying to regulations, or meeting environmental objectives.

To be really efficient and effective, the organization can manage its way of doing things by systemizing it. Nothing important is left out. Everyone is clear about who is responsible for doing what, when, how, why and where. Management system standards provide the organization with an international state-of-the-art model to follow. Large organizations, or ones with complicated processes, could not function well without management systems.

Companies in such fields as aerospace, automobiles, defense, or health care devices have been operating management systems for years.

The ISO 9001 and ISO 14001 management system standards now make these successful practices available for all organizations.

Both ISO 9001 and ISO 14001 concern the way an organization goes about its work. They are not product standards. They are not service standards. They are process standards. They can be used by product manufacturers and service providers. Processes affect final products or services.

ISO 9001 gives the requirements for what the organization must do to manage processes affecting quality of its products and services.

ISO 14001 gives the requirements for what the organization must do manage processes affecting the impact of its activities on the environment.

Certification and Registration

Certification is known in some countries as registration. It means that an independent, external body has audited an organization's management system and verified that it conforms to the requirements specified in the standard (ISO 9001 or ISO 14001). ISO does not carry out certification and does not issue or approve certificates,

Accreditation

Accreditation is like certification of the certification body. It means the formal approval by a specialized body - an accreditation body - that a certification body is competent to carry out ISO 9001:2008 or ISO 14001:2004 certification in specified business sectors. Certificates issued by accredited certification bodies - and known as accredited certificates - may be perceived on the market as having increased credibility. ISO does not carry out or approve accreditations.

Certification not a Requirement

Certification is not a requirement of ISO 9001 or ISO 14001. The organization can implement and benefit from an ISO 9001 or ISO 14001 system without having it certified. The organization can implement them for the internal benefits without spending money on a certification programme.

Certification is a Business Decision

Certification is a decision to be taken for business reasons: if it is a contractual, regulatory, or market requirement, If it meets customer preferences it is part of a risk management programme, or if it will motivate staff by setting a clear goal.

ISO does not certify

ISO does not carry out ISO 9001 or ISO 14001 certification. ISO does not issue certificates. ISO does not accredit, approve or control the certification bodies.

ISO develops standards and guides to encourage good practice in accreditation and certification.

The ISO 9000 family

ISO 9001 is the standard that gives the requirements for a quality management system. ISO 9001:2008 is the latest, improved version. It is the only standard in the ISO 9000 family that can be used for certification. There are 16 other standards in the family that can help an organization on specific aspects such as performance improvement, auditing, training.

The ISO 14000 family

ISO 14001 is the standard that gives the requirements for an environmental management system.ISO 14001:2004 is the latest, improved version. It is the only standard in the ISO 14000 family that can be used for certification. The ISO 14000 family includes 21 other standards that can help an organization specific aspect such as auditing, environmental labelling, life cycle analysis.

Benefits of ISO 9001 and ISO 14001

(i) International, expert consensus on state-of-the-art practices for quality and environmental management.
(ii) Common language for dealing with customers and suppliers worldwide in B2B.
(iii) Increase efficiency and effectiveness.
(iv) Model for continual improvement.
(v) Model for satisfying customers and other stakeholders.
(vi) Build quality into products and services from design onwards.
(vii) Address environmental concerns of customers and public, and comply with government regulations.
(viii) Integrate with global economy.
(ix) Sustainable business
(x) Unifying base for industry sectors
(xi) Qualify suppliers for global supply chains
(xii) Technical support for regulations
(xiii) Transfer of good practice to developing countries
(xiv) Tools for new economic players
(xv) Regional integration
(xvi) Facilitate rise of services

ISO Registration Process (Steps for Registration)

The ISO Registration Process comes after your company's ISO 9001 audit. The purpose of registering your company is to show that you've met the requirements. And to do this effectively, you will need to follow eight essential steps.

1. **Finding an ISO 9001 Registrar**

   It is needed to search for an ISO registrar during the 2 to 3 months your company is still building its quality system. Search the ANSI-ASQ National Accreditation Board (ANAB) to select the registrar.

   Registrars must meet the requirements of the ISO Accreditation Bodies. These requirements include things such as independence; Registrars cannot consult for instance. This system ensures uniformity in the registration process.

   Accreditation Bodies maintain directories of the Registrar organizations that they accredit. These directories are available on their websites. We can normally find these websites by doing a search on the Accreditation Body's name or initials.

   A directory of registrars in the U.S. can also be found at the ANSI-ASQ National Accreditation Board website which offers access to a searchable database of accredited registrars in the United States.

   In Canada, contact the Standards Council of Canada for a list of registrars. All other countries should consult the accreditation authority or member body for their country. Consult the ISO website for a complete list of ISO Member bodies.

2. **Selecting an ISO Registrar**

   Select a registrar that has experience within the scope category of your specific industry, which you can also find on the ANAB site. Keep in mind accreditation, scheduling issues, fees and comfort level when selecting the registrar right for you.

   Registrar qualifications are a key consideration. As you research Registrars, you will notice that some appear to be very limited in scope just based on their names. Registrars must be accredited in a particular industrial sector in order for them to be able to certify a company in that sector. Some Registrars are accredited in several if not all sectors; others specialize in certain sectors. The best approach to evaluating a Registrar's qualifications for your industrial sector is to contact the Registrar.

   After qualifications, price is always a concern. Be sure to evaluate the total cost including expenses, fees and the cost of surveillance.

Probably as important as price, within limits of course, is the overall experience a client gets with a registrar. Important areas to consider are the interpersonal skills of the auditors; the office support and ability to get questions answered; are the audits a value-added experience, will the Registrar work with you, how flexible are they in adjusting dates – how many weeks notice.

3. **Creating an ISO Application**

A company and a registrar will agree on the application contract. This is an important step of the ISO Registration Process because it defines the rights and obligations of both parties, and includes liability issues, confidentiality and access rights.

4. **Conducting a Quality Document Review**

The registrar will require a copy of your quality manual and procedures to verify that all the requirements of the standard are addressed. The ISO Registration Process is not a quick process, be sure to allow 2-4 weeks in advance for the registrar to fully review all of the necessary documents.

5. **Determining Preassessment Need**

Though optional, this 2-4 week initial review of the system identifies any significant omissions or weaknesses. It saves time and allows the registrar to assess any issues and resolve logistics before the actual assessment audit.

The Preassessment is an initial review of your Quality Management System to identify any significant omissions or weaknesses in the system and provide your organization an opportunity to correct any deficiencies before the regular registration assessment is conducted.

6. **Issuing an ISO Assessment**

During the audit, or physical onsite inspection of procedures in action, the auditors will issue findings if they assess anything that doesn't meet requirements, or nonconformities. The length of this step of the ISO Registration Process will depend on the scope of the audit and the size your organization.

In general, the flow of activities during the audit is as follows:

1. Opening Meeting. An introduction of the audit team and key personnel in your company. The scope and general approach to the audit is discussed. This is also the time to question anything that is unclear in the audit schedule and communicate any last minute changes to the system or schedule.

2. Brief tour of the facility. Keep it brief, the auditors just want to get a general feel for the layout and processes involved. This may also be done at the preassessment.
3. Additional review of documents. Audit team members review documentation for areas they will audit.
4. Examination. The audit is conducted, personnel are interviewed, and objective evidence is collected to show the system has been effectively implemented.
5. Daily review. At the end of each day or the beginning of the next, the audit team reviews any issues identified during the assessment. Potential findings or nonconformities may be clarified at this time.
6. Closing Meeting. The audit team states their conclusions regarding the audit and presents any findings or nonconformities that were identified along with any observations they may have.
7. Audit Report issued. Within a few weeks of the audit, the Registrar issues the audit report. The report generally restates what was discussed in the closing meeting.

During the audit, if the auditors find anything that does not meet with the requirements of the ISO standard or that does not meet the requirements of your procedures, they determine the severity and issue a finding. Audit findings are usually called nonconformities and fall into one of two categories depending on severity.

A Minor Nonconformance deals with minor infractions of procedures or minor failures of the system in meeting the ISO 9001:2008 requirements. These will not hold up your registration.

A Major Nonconformance deals with issues where nonconforming product is likely to reach the customer or where there is a breakdown in the Quality System that results in the system not being effective in meeting the requirements of the standard. This will hold up your registration.

The primary difference to you between a major and minor nonconformance is that your registration cannot proceed until all major nonconformities are closed and verified by the Registrar. This usually involves a re-audit of the involved areas and, of course, the associated costs. Minor nonconformities require a corrective action plan and they are closed at the first surveillance.

ISO Auditors

Auditors work for or contract to Registrars to perform registration assessments and surveillances. They are the "front line" in the process. The Registrars are responsible for ensuring Auditors meet qualification requirements. Their requirements include training in auditing, ISO 9001 training, and at least one member of the audit team must have experience in the industrial sector of the company being audited.

Verify credentials of a person claims to be certified as an ISO 9000 lead auditor, ask to see proof of his or her certification. Make sure the certification is current by checking the expiration date. Facts about ASQ's certification are available via the ASQ website.

Auditors collect the objective evidence demonstrating the effectiveness (or lack thereof) of the company's quality management system and make registration recommendations to the Registrar. The Registrar has the ultimate decision, however.

7. **Completing ISO 9001 Registration**

   After all of the findings are put into the ISO audit report and nonconformities are addressed, your company has the option to register as ISO 9001 conformant. You will receive a certificate and can also be listed in a register, which the company can use to publicize its registration and use in advertising.

8. **Checking with Surveillance Audits**

   To ensure that the system is maintained and that changes don't result in deficiencies in the system, registrars perform regular surveillances of the system. Over the three-year period of your certificate, auditors will perform one full and two partial checks of your system.

National Accreditation Board for Testing and Calibration Laboratories (NABL)

NABL is an autonomous society providing Accreditation (Recognition) of Technical competence of a testing, calibration, medical laboratory and Proficiency testing provider (PTP) and Reference Material Producer (RMP). NABL stands for National Accreditation Board For Testing And Calibration Laboratories. NABL has agreements with ILAC (International Laboratory Accreditation Conference) and APLAC (Asia Pacific Laboratory Accreditation Cooperation). These are especially valuable for International recognition and mutual acceptance of test results. In short accreditation has worldwide acceptance.

NABL specifies the general requirements for the competence to carry out tests and calibrations, including sampling. It covers testing and calibration performed using standard methods, non-standard methods, and laboratory-developed methods.

NABL is an autonomous body under the aegis of Department of Science & Technology, Government of India, and is registered under the Societies Act. It is only one of its kinds that assess laboratories in India for quality and consistency in the results. The concept of Laboratory Accreditation was developed to provide a means for third party certification of the competence of laboratories to perform specific type(s) of testing.

NABL Vision

To be the world's leading accreditation body and to enhance stakeholders' confidence in its services.

NABL Mission

To strengthen the accreditation system accepted across the globe by providing high quality, value driven services, fostering APLAC/ILAC MRA, empanelling competent assessors, creating awareness among the stake holders, initiating new programs supporting accreditation activities and pursuing organizational excellence.

Benefits of NABL Accreditation

- Potential increase in business due to enhanced customer confidence and satisfaction.
- Savings in terms of time and money due to reduction or elimination of the need for re-testing.
- Better control of laboratory operations and feedback to laboratories as to whether they have sound Quality Assurance System and are technically competent.
- Increase of confidence in Testing / Calibration data and personnel performing work.
- Customers can search and identify the laboratories accredited by NABL for their specific requirements from the directory of Accredited Laboratories.
- Users of accredited laboratories will enjoy greater access for their products, in both domestic and international markets, when tested by accredited laboratories.

Types of Laboratory can seek Accreditation

- Laboratories undertaking any sort of testing or calibration in the specified fields.
- Private or government laboratories.

- Small operations to large multi-field laboratories.
- Site facilities, temporary field operations and mobile laboratories.

10 Step Approach to Accreditation

- Awareness Training
- Quality Policy & Objectives Finalization
- Gap Analysis
- Documentation / Process Design
- Documentation / Process Implementation
- Internal Audit
- Management Review Meeting
- Shadow Audit
- Corrective –Preventive Actions
- Final Certification Audit

Step 1: Awareness Training

Separate training sessions for top management, middle management and junior level management.

Creates a motivating environment throughout the organization for ISO 17025 implementation.

Step 2: Quality Policy & Objectives

Work shop with top management on development of quality policy.

Work shop with top management and middle level functional management on development of quality objectives.

Step 3: Gap Analysis

Understanding of all the operations of the organization.

Development of process map for the activities of the organization.

Comparing existing operations with requirements of ISO 17025:2005 standard.

Step 4: Documentation / Process Design

Quality Manual

Functional Procedures

Work Instructions

System Procedures

Formats

Step 5: Documentation / Process Implementation

Workshop on process / document implementation as per ISO 17025 requirements.

Departmental / Individual assistance in implementing the new processes / documents.

Step 6: Internal Audit

Internal Audit Training & Examination (Optional).

Successful employees / we carry out internal audit of the organization covering all the departments and operations.

Suggest corrective and preventive actions for improvements in each of the audited departments.

Step 7: Management Review Meeting

Quality Policy & Objectives

Results of internal audit

Results of supplier evaluation

Results of customer complaints

Results of customer feedback etc.

Step 8: Shadow Audit

A replica of final certification audit.

Finds degree of compliance with ISO 17025 standard.

Gives an idea to the employees about the conduct of the final certification audit.

Step 9: Corrective –Preventive Actions

On the basis of shadow audit conducted in the last step, all the non-conformities will be assigned corrective and preventive actions.

A check will ensure that all the NCs are closed and the organization is ready for the final certification audit.

Step 10: Final Certification Audit

Upon completion of various stages of accreditation audit, the audit, your organization will be aw.

CHPATER - 7

Validation in cGMP (Process Validation)

Learning Objectives

To learn about:

- Concept and Definitions of Validation
- Need and Scope of Validation
- Importance of Validation
- Planning for Validation
- Validation Master Plan (VMP)
- Advantages of Validation (Assurance of Quality, Process Optimization, Reduction of Quality Cost and Safety)
- Types of Validation
- Prospective Validation
- Concurrent Validation
- Retrospective Validation
- Re Validation
- Basic concepts of Process Validation
- Installation Qualification (IQ)
- Operational Qualification (OQ)
- Performance Qualification (PQ)
- Re Qualification
- Prerequisites of Process Validation
- Reasons for Process Validation
- Benefits of Process Validation
- Stages of Process Validation
- Validation Protocol
- Validation Master Plan
- Validation Report
- Documentation

Introduction

The prime objective of any pharmaceutical plant is to manufacture products of requisite attribute and quality consistently, at the lowest possible cost. Although validation studies have been conducted in the pharmaceutical industry for a long time, there is an ever increasing interest in validation owing to their industry's greater emphasis in recent years on quality assurance program and is fundamental to an efficient production operation.

Validation is a concept that has evolved in united states in 1978.The concept of validation has expanded through the years to embrace a wide range of activities from analytical methods used for the quality control of drug substances and drug products to computerized systems for clinical trials, labeling or process control, Validation is founded on, but not prescribed by regulatory requirements and is best viewed as an important and integral part of Cgmp.

The concept of validation was first proposed by two FDA officials, Ted Byers and Bud Loftus, in the mid 1970's in order to improve the quality of pharmaceuticals .It was proposed in direct response to several problems in the sterility of large volume parenteral market. The first validation activities were focused on the processes involved in making these products, but quickly spread to associated process of pharmaceutical.

U.S.F.D.A. was the pioneer in advocating the concept of process validation, but till 29th September 1978 the definition of process validation did not appear in any part of literature of U.S.F.D.A. no cGMP regulations talked anything about process validation.

Definitions European commission

1991 –Validation-"Act of proving, in accordance of GMPs that Any…" process actually leads to expected results.

2000 -"Documented evidence that the process, operated within established Parameters, can perform effectively and reproducibly to produce a Medicinal product meeting its predetermined specifications and quality attributes".

US FDA Definition

"Process validation is establishing documented evidence which provides a high degree of assurance that a specified process will consistently produce a product meeting its pre-determined specifications and quality characteristics."

ICH Definition

"Process Validation is the means of ensuring and providing documentary evidence that processes within their specified design parameters are capable of repeatedly and reliably producing a finished product of the required quality."

WHO Definition

"The documented act of proving that any procedure, process, equipment, material, activity or system actually leads to expected result."

Need of Pharmaceutical Validation

Validation is an integral part of quality assurance; it involves the systematic study of systems, facilities and processes aimed at determining whether they perform their intended functions adequately and consistently as specified. A validated process is one which has been demonstrated to provide a high degree of assurance that uniform batches will be produced that meet the required specifications and has therefore been formally approved. Validation in itself does not improve processes but confirms that the processes have been properly developed and are under control.

Scope of Validation

Pharmaceutical Validation is a vast area of work and it practically covers every aspect of pharmaceutical processing activities, hence defining the Scope of Validation becomes a really difficult task. However, a systematic look at the pharmaceutical operations will point out at least the following areas for pharmaceutical validation;

- Analytical
- Instrument Calibration
- Process Utility services
- Raw materials
- Packaging materials
- Equipment
- Facilities
- Manufacturing operations
- Product Design
- Cleaning
- Operators

Importance of Validation

- Assurance of quality
- Time bound
- Process optimization
- Reduction of quality cost
- Nominal mix-ups, and bottle necks
- Minimal batch failures, improved efficiently and productivity
- Reduction in rejections
- Increased output
- Avoidance of capital expenditures
- Fewer complaints about process related failures
- Reduced testing in process and in finished goods
- More rapid and reliable start-up of new equipments
- Easier scale-up form development work
- Easier maintenance of equipment
- Improved employee awareness of processes
- More rapid automation
- Government regulation (Compliance with validation requirements is necessary for obtaining approval to manufacture and to introduce new products)

Planning for Validation

All validation activities should be planned. The key elements of a validation programme should be clearly defined and documented in a validation master plan (VMP) or equivalent documents.

- The VMP should be a summary document, which is brief, concise and clear.
- The VMP should contain data on at least the following:
  - Validation policy.
  - Organizational structure of validation activities.
  - Summary of facilities, systems, equipment and processes to be validated.
  - Documentation format: The format to be used for protocols and reports.
  - Planning and scheduling.

- o Change control.
- o Reference to existing document.
- o In case of large projects, it may be necessary to create separate validation master plans.

Four Major Advantages of Validation Namely Assurance of Quality

Validation is an extension of the concepts of quality assurance since close control of the process is necessary to assure product quality and it is not possible to control a process properly without thorough knowledge of the capabilities of that process without validated and controlled processes, it is impossible to produce quality products consistently. End product testing, in the absence of validation, gives little assurance of quality for variety reasons, among which are

- Very limited sample size.
- The limited number of tests performed on a sample. For example, it is impractical to test for all potential impurities or contaminants.
- The limited sensitivity of the test

Process Optimization

The optimization of a process for maximum efficiency, while maintaining quality standards, is a consequence of validation. Literal meaning of word to optimize is "To make as effective, perfect or useful as possible". The optimization of the facility, equipment, systems, and processes results in a product that meets quality requirements at the lowest cost.

Reduction of Quality Costs

Quality costs are divided in to four categories. They are:

- Preventive costs.
- Appraisal costs.
- Internal failure costs.
- External failure costs.

Of internal failure costs: Any validated and controlled process will result in fewer internal failures like

- Fewer rejects
- Reworks
- Re-tests
- Re-inspection

Process validation makes it possible to do the job right the first time. Also, a scientifically studied and controlled process makes it unlikely that defective products will be dispatched to market thus no recalls or market complaints.

Safety

Validation can also result in increased operation safety. e.g.: gauges used on equipment that designed to operate at certain temperature and pressures must be reliable i.e. they must be calibrated.

Types/Methods of Validation

Prospective Validation

It is defined as the established documented evidence that a system does what it purports to do based on a pre- planned protocol. This validation usually carried out prior to distribution either of a new product or a product made under a revised manufacturing process. Performed on at least three successive production-sizes (Consecutive batches).

In Prospective Validation, the validation protocol is executed before the process is put into commercial use. During the product development phase, the production process should be categorized into individual steps. Each step should be evaluated on the basis of experience or theoretical considerations to determine the critical parameters that may affect the quality of the finished product. A series of experiment should be designed to determine the criticality of these factors. Each experiment should be planned and documented fully in an authorized protocol.

All equipment, production environment and the analytical testing methods to be used should have been fully validated. Master batch documents can be prepared only after the critical parameters of the process have been identified and machine settings, component specifications and environmental conditions have been determined.

Using this defined process a series of batches should be produced. In theory, the number of process runs carried out and observations made should be sufficient to allow the normal extent of variation and trends to be established to provide sufficient data for evaluation. It is generally considered acceptable that three consecutive batches/runs within the finally agreed parameters, giving product of the desired quality would constitute a proper validation of the process.

In practice, it may take some considerable time to accumulate these data. Some considerations should be exercised when selecting the process validation strategy. Amongst these should be the use of different lots of active raw materials and major excipients, batches produced on different shifts, the use of different equipment and facilities dedicated for commercial production, operating range of the critical processes, and a thorough analysis of the process data in case of Requalification and Revalidation.

During the processing of the validation batches, extensive sampling and testing should be performed on the product at various stages and should be documented comprehensively. Detailed testing should also be done on the final product in its package.

Upon completion of the review, recommendations should be made on the extent of monitoring and the in- process controls necessary for routine production. These should be incorporated into the Batch manufacturing and packaging record or into appropriate standard operating procedures.

Limits, frequencies and action to be taken in the event of the limits being exceeded should be specified.

Prospective validation should include, but not be limited to the following:

- Short description of the process.
- Summary of the critical processing steps to be investigated.
- List of the equipment/facilities to be used (including measuring, monitoring/recording equipment) together with its calibration status.
- Finished product specifications for release.
- List of analytical methods, as appropriate.
- Proposed in-process controls with acceptance criteria.
- Additional testing to be carried out, with acceptance criteria and analytical validation, as appropriate.
- Sampling plan.
- Methods for recording and evaluating results.
- Functions and responsibilities.
- Proposed timetable.

Batches made for process validation should be the same size as the intended Industrial scale batches. If it is intended that validation batches be sold or supplied, the conditions under which they are produced should comply fully with the requirements of Good Manufacturing Practice, including the satisfactory outcome of the validation exercise and the marketing authorization.

Concurrent Validation

It is similar to prospective, except the operating firm will sell the product during the qualification runs, to the public at its market price, and also similar to retrospective validation.

- This validation involves in-process monitoring of critical processing steps and product testing. This helps to generate and documented evidence to show that the production process is in a state of control.
- In exceptional circumstances it may be acceptable not to complete a validation programme before routine production starts.
- The decision to carry out concurrent validation must be justified, documented and approved by authorized personnel.
- Documentation requirements for concurrent validation are the same as specified for prospective validation.

Retrospective Validation

It is defined as the established documented evidence that a system does what it purports to do on the review and analysis of historical information. This is achieved by the review of the historical manufacturing testing data to prove that the process has always remained in control. This type of validation of a process for a product already in distribution.

Retrospective validation is only acceptable for well- established processes and will be inappropriate where there have been recent changes in the composition of the product, operating procedures or equipment.

Validation of such processes should be based on historical data. The steps involved require the preparation of a specific protocol and the reporting of the results of the data review, leading to a conclusion and a recommendation.

The source of data for this validation should include, but not be limited to batch processing and packaging records, process control charts, maintenance logbooks, records of personnel changes, process capability studies, finished product data, including trend cards and storage stability results.

Batches selected for retrospective validation should be representative of all batches made during the review period, including any batches that failed to meet the specifications, and should be sufficient in number to demonstrate process consistency. Additional testing of retained samples may be needed to obtain the necessary amount or type of data to retrospectively validate the process.

For retrospective validation, generally data from ten to thirty consecutive batches should be examined to access process consistency, but fewer batches may be examined if justified.

Some of the essential elements for Retrospective Validation

Batches manufactured for a defined period (minimum of 10 last consecutive batches). Number of lots released per year.

- Batch size/strength/manufacturer/year/period.
- Master manufacturing/packaging documents.
- Current specifications for active materials/finished products.
- List of process deviations, corrective actions and changes to manufacturing documents.
- Data for stability testing for several batches.

Revalidation

Re-validation provides the evidence that changes in a process and/or the process environment that are introduced do not adversely affect process characteristics and product quality. Documentation requirements will be the same as for the initial validation of the process.

Facilities, systems, equipment and processes, including cleaning, should be periodically evaluated to confirm that they remain valid. Where no significant changes have been made to the validated status, a review with evidence that facilities, systems, equipment and processes meet the prescribed requirements fulfils the need for revalidation.

Revalidation becomes necessary in certain situations. Some of the changes that require validation are as follows:

- Changes in raw materials (physical properties such as density, viscosity, particle size distribution and moisture etc that may affect the process or product).
- Changes in the source of active raw material manufacturer.
- Changes in packaging material (primary container/closure system)
- Changes in the process (e.g., mixing time, drying temperatures and batch size)
- Changes in the equipment (e.g., addition of automatic detection system). Changes of equipment which involve the replacement of equipment on a "like for like" basis would not normally require re-validation except that this new equipment must be qualified.

Changes in the plant/facility.

A decision not to perform revalidation studies must be fully justified and documented.

Basic Concept of Process Validation

Pharmaceutical Process Validation is the most important and recognized parameters of cGMPs. The requirement of process validation appears of the quality system (QS) regulation. The goal of a quality system is to consistently produce products that are fit for their intended use.

Process validation is a key element in assuring that these principles and goal are met. The process validation is standardization of the validation documents that must be submitted with the submission file for marketing authorization. The process validation is intended to assist manufacturers in understanding quality management system (QMS) requirements concerning process validation and has general applicability to manufacturing process. According to FDA,

Assurance of product quality is derived from careful and systemic attention to a number of importance factors, including selection of quality process through in-process and end product testing.

The basic principle for validation may be stated as follows:

Installation Qualification (IQ)

Establishing by objective evidence that all key aspects of the process equipment and ancillary system installation adhere to the manufacturer's approved specification and that the recommendation of the supplier of the equipment are suitably considered.

IQ considerations are:

- Equipment design features (i.e. material of construction clean ability, etc.)
- Installation conditions (wiring, utility, functionality, etc.)
- Calibration, preventative maintenance, cleaning schedules.
- Safety features.
- Supplier documentation, prints, drawings and manuals.
- Software documented.
- Spare parts list.
- Environmental conditions (such as clean room requirements, temperature, and humidity).

Operational Qualification (OQ)

Establishing by objective evidence process control limits and action levels which result in product that all predetermined requirements.

OQ considerations include:

- Process control limits (time, temperature, pressure, line speed, setup conditions, etc.)
- Software parameters.
- Raw material specifications
- Process operating procedures.
- Material handling requirements.
- Process change control.
- Training.
- Short term stability and capability of the process, (latitude studies or control charts).
- Potential failure modes, action levels and worst-case conditions.
- The use of statistically valid techniques such as screening experiments to optimize the process can be used during this phase.

Performance Qualification (PQ)

Establishing by objective evidence that the process, under anticipated conditions, consistently produces a product which meets all predetermined requirements.

PQ considerations include:

- Actual product and process parameters and procedures established in OQ.
- Acceptability of the product.
- Assurance of process capability as established in OQ.
- Process repeatability, long term process stability.

Re – Qualification

Modification to, or relocation of equipment should follow satisfactory review and authorization of the documented change proposal through the change control procedure. This formal review should include consideration of re qualification of the equipment. Minor changes or changes having no direct impact on final or in-process product quality should be handled through the documentation system of the preventive maintenance program.

Prerequisite of Process Validation

- Process Development Designee shall review the product development report, data from pilot scale, scale up batch and proposed master formula document of product intended for manufacturing.
- Process Development Designee shall review/ensure the availability analytical method transfer report to the plant and plant preparedness for conducting validation testing and routine testing; function shall co-ordinate with QC/QA in this regard.
- Process Development Designee shall prepare commercial/exhibit batch production and control records which include the operational limits and overall strategy for process control based on development report.
- The Process Validation is performed after the facility, utility, and equipment, and laboratory test methods have been validated and released for process validation activities. Where compendia method is used only limited analytical method validation shall be conducted.
- All raw material and packaging material specification shall be from approved vendors and shall be approved by quality control.
- All the equipment and instrument to be utilized are calibrated and preventive maintenance programs are in place.
- Relevant SOPs are in place and training is completed on equipment, operation, manufacturing instruction and sampling strategy.
- Key process steps and process variables are identified and their operating ranges have been established.
- All the master formula, manufacturing instruction, packaging instruction, testing procedure and specification shall be approved before execution of process validation batches.
- The cleaning of the area and equipment has been completed prior to the initiation of process validation.

The validation team and operational team shall be trained from process engineer

Strategy for Industrial Process Validation of Solid Dosage Forms

The strategy selected for process validation should be simple and straightforward. The following five points gives strategy for process validation.

- The use of different lots of raw materials should be included. i.e., active drug substance and major excipients.

- Batches should be run in succession and on different days and shifts (the latter condition, if appropriate).
- Batches should be manufactured in the equipment and facilities designated for eventual commercial production.
- Critical process variables should be set within their operating ranges and should not exceed their upper and lower control limits during process operation. Output responses should be well within finished product specifications.
- Failure to meet the requirements of the Validation protocol with respect to process input and output control should be subjected to process requalification and subsequent revalidation.

Process Validation within the Quality Management System

Process validation is part of the integrated requirements of a quality management system. It is conducted in the context of a system including design and development control, quality assurance, process control, and corrective and preventive action. The product should be design robustly enough to withstand variations in the manufacturing process and the manufacturing process should be capable and stable to assure continued safe products that perform adequately. Corrective actions often identify inadequate processes/process validations. Each corrective action applied to a manufacturing process should include the consideration for conducting process validation/ revalidation.

Reason for Process Validation

The possible reason of performing process validation may include:

- New product or existing products as per SUPAC changes.
- Change in site of manufacturing.
- Change in batch size.
- Change in equipment.
- Change in process existing products.
- Change in composition or components.
- Change in the critical control parameters.
- Change in vendor of API or critical excipient.
- Change in specification on input material.
- Abnormal trends in quality parameters of product through review during Annual Product Review (APR).
- Trend of Out of Specification (OOS) or Out of Trend (OOT) in consecutive batches.

Benefits of Process Validation

- Consistent through output.
- Reduction in rejections and reworks.
- Reduction in utility cost.
- Avoidance of capital expenditures.
- Fewer complaints about process related failure.
- Reduced testing in process and finished goods.
- More rapid and accurate investigations into process deviation.
- More rapid and reliable start-up of new equipment.
- Easier scale-up from development work.
- Easier maintenance of equipment.
- Improve employee awareness of processes.
- More rapid automation.

Stages of Process Validation

Process Validation is defined as the collection and evaluation of data, from the process design stage through commercial production, which establishes scientific evidence that a process is capable of consistently delivering quality product. Process Validation involves a series of activities taking place over the lifecycle of the product and process. The activities relating to validation studies may be classified into three stages:

Stage 1 – Process Design

"Focusing exclusively on qualification efforts without also understanding the manufacturing process is defined during this stage based on knowledge gained through development and scale-up activities. It covers all activities relating to product research and development, formulation, pilot batch studies, scale-up studies, transfer of technology to commercial scale batches, establishing stability conditions, storage and handling of in-process and finished dosage forms, equipment qualification, installation qualification, master production documents, operational qualification, process capability. Also, this is the stage in which the establishment of a strategy for process control is taking place using accumulation knowledge and understanding of the process."

Stage 2 – Process Qualification

During this stage, the process design is evaluated to determine if the process is capable of reproducible commercial manufacturing. It confirms that all established limits of the Critical Process Parameters are valid and that satisfactory products can be produced even under "worst case" conditions. GMP compliant procedures must be followed in this stage and successful completion of this stage is necessary before commercial distribution of a product.

There are two aspect of Process Qualification:

- Design of Facilities and Qualification of Equipment and Utilities
    - Proper design of manufacturing facility is desired under 21 CFR part 211, subpart C, of the cGMP regulation on Buildings and Facilities.
    - Activities performed to assure proper facility design and that the equipment and utilities are suitable for their intended use and perform properly.
- Process Performance Qualification

  "Criteria and process performance indicators that allow for a science and risk-based decision about the ability of the process to consistently produce quality products".
    - Part of the planning for stage 2 involves defining performance criteria and deciding what data to collect when, how much data, and appropriate analysis of the data.
    - Likely consist of planned comparisons and evaluations of some combination of process measures as well as in-process and trial product attributes.
    - Manufacturer must scientifically determine suitable criteria and justify it.
    - Objective measures, wherever possible.
    - May be possible to leverage earlier study data if relevant to the commercial scale.

Stage 3 – Continued Process Verification

Ongoing assurance is gained during routine production that the process remains in a state of control. The validation maintenance stage requires frequent review of all process related documents, including validation audit reports to assure that there have been no changes, deviations, failures, modifications to the production process, and that all SOPs have been followed, including change control procedures.

A successful validation program depends on the knowledge and understanding and the approach to control manufacturing processes. These include the source of variation, the limitation of the detection of the variation, and the attributes susceptible of the variation.

Primary packing will be done for individual packing, the process validation protocol shall be clearly state the variable(s) which impact the integrity of the primary pack and set parameters range, primary packing is mostly change part specific and it is mandatory for all new products.

For existing products it shall be performed based on matrix approach w.r.t pocket size for blister /strip and different size of HDPE bottles/containers.

The activity starts with documenting the change part number and establishing the proven acceptance range-

PAR for the machine set parameters

∴ Sealing temp/speed in blister and strip packing machine, for dry syrups /sterile products speed and sealing torque, for tablets capsules bulk packed in HDPE bottles, the speed and induction sealing, power voltage and conveyer speed for topically filled in collapsible tubes, speed and crimping quality PAR shall be established for each configuration.

Validation Protocol

Detailed protocols for performing validations are essential to ensure that the process is adequately validated. Process validation protocols should include the following elements:

- Objectives, scope of coverage of the validation study.
- Validation team membership, their qualifications and responsibilities.
- Type of validation: prospective, concurrent, retrospective, re-validation.
- Number and selection of batches to be on the validation study.
- A list of all equipment to be used; their normal and worst case operating parameters.
- Outcome of IQ, OQ for critical equipment.
- Requirements for calibration of all measuring devices.
- Critical process parameters and their respective tolerances.
- Process variables and attributes with probable risk and prevention shall be captured.
- Description of the processing steps: copy of the master documents for the product.
- Sampling points, stages of sampling, methods of sampling, sampling plans.
- Statistical tools to be used in the analysis of data.
- Training requirements for the processing operators.

- Validated test methods to be used in in process testing and for the finished product.
- Specifications for raw and packaging materials and test methods.
- Forms and charts to be used for documenting results.
- Format for presentation of results, documenting conclusions and for approval of study results.

Validation Master Plan

The validation master plan should provide an overview of the entire validation operation, its organizational structure, its content and planning. The main elements of it being the list/inventory of the items to be validated and the planning schedule.

All validation activities relating to critical technical operations, relevant to product and process controls within a firm should be included in the validation master plan.

It should comprise all prospective, concurrent and retrospective validations as well as revalidation.

The Validation Master Plan should be a summary document and should therefore be brief, concise and clear. It should not repeat information documented elsewhere but should refer to existing documents such as policy documents,

SOP's and validation protocols and reports. The format and content should include:

- Introduction: validation policy, scope, location and schedule.
- Organizational structure: personnel responsibilities.
- Plant/process/product description: rational for inclusions or exclusions and extent of validation.
- Specific process considerations that are critical and those requiring extra attention.
- List of products/ processes/ systems to be validated, summarized in a matrix format, validation approach.
- Re-validation activities, actual status and
- Key acceptance criteria.
- Documentation format.
- Reference to the required SOP's.
- Time plans of each validation project and sub-project.

Validation Report

A written report should be available after completion of the validation. If found acceptable, it should be approved and authorized (signed and dated). The report should include at least the following:

- Title and objective of study.
- Reference to protocol.
- Details of material.
- Equipment.
- Programmes and cycles used.
- Details of procedures and test methods.
- Results (compared with acceptance criteria).
- Recommendations on the limit and criteria to be applied on future basis.

Documentation

A written protocol should be established that specifies how qualification and validation will be conducted. The protocol should be reviewed and approved. The protocol should specify critical steps and acceptance criteria.

A report that cross-references the qualification and/or validation protocol should be prepared, summarizing the results obtained, commenting on any deviations observed, and drawing the necessary conclusions, including recommending changes necessary to correct deficiencies. Any changes to the plan as defined in the protocol should be documented with appropriate justification.

After completion of a satisfactory qualification, a format release for the next step in qualification and validation should be made as a written authorization.

CHPATER - 8

Good Manufacturing Practices (GMP)-Part 1

(Introduction Summary, Organization, Personnel and Premises)

Learning Objectives

To learn about:

- History of GMP
- Quality Management and GMP
- Definitions of various terms in GMP
- Summary of GMP guidelines
- Components of GMP
- Organization and Personnel
- Key Personnel
- Responsibilities of Head of Production
- Responsibilities of Head of Quality Control
- Training
- Personal Hygiene
- Premises
- Ancillary Areas
- Storage Areas
- Weighing Areas
- Production Areas
- Quality Control Areas
- Sanitation and Hygiene

Introduction and History

The first WHO draft text on good manufacturing practices (GMP) was prepared in 1967 by a group of consultants at the request of the Twentieth World Health Assembly (resolution WHA20.34). It was subsequently submitted to the Twenty-first World Health Assembly under the title "Draft requirements for good manufacturing practice in the manufacture and quality control of drugs and pharmaceutical specialties" and was accepted.

The revised text was discussed by the WHO Expert committee on specifications for Pharmaceutical Preparations in 1968 and published as an annex to its twenty-second report. The text was then reproduced (with some revisions) in 1971 in the supplement to the second edition of The International Pharmacopoeia.

In 1969, when the World Health Assembly recommended the first version of the WHO Certification Scheme on the Quality of Pharmaceutical Products Moving in International Commerce in resolution WHA22.50, it accepted at the same time the GMP text as an integral part of the scheme. Revised versions of both the certification scheme and the GMP text were adopted in 1975 by resolution WHA28.65. Since then, the Certification Scheme has been extended to include the certification of:-veterinary products administered to food-producing animals;-starting materials for use in dosage forms, when they are subject to control by legislation in both the exporting Member state and the importing Member state;-information on safety and efficacy (resolution WHA41.18,1988).

In 1992, the revised draft requirements for GMP were presented in three parts, of which only parts One and Two are reproduced in this document (1).

Quality Management and GMP

"Quality management in the drug industry: philosophy and essential elements" outlines the general concepts of quality assurance as well as the principal components or subsystems of GMP, which are joint responsibilities of top management and production and quality control management. These include hygiene, validation, self-inspection, personnel, premises, equipment, materials and documentation.

"Good practices in production" (section 16) and "Good practices in quality control" (section 17), provide guidance on actions to be taken separately by production and by quality control personnel for the implementation of the general principles of quality assurance.

These two parts were subsequently supplemented by further guidelines which are integral parts of these good manufacturing practices for pharmaceutical products. All these texts are available on the web page of the World Health Organization.

Considerable developments in GMP have taken place in the intervening years, and important national and international documents, including new revisions, have appeared (2, 3, 4, 5). Thus, the necessity to revise the main principles and incorporate the concept of validation.

Definitions

The definitions given below apply to the terms used in this guide. They may have different meanings in other contexts.

Active Pharmaceutical Ingredient (Api)

Any substance or mixture of substances intended to be used in the manufacture of a pharmaceutical dosage form and that, when so used, becomes an active ingredient of that pharmaceutical dosage form. Such substances are intended to furnish pharmacological activity or other direct effect in the diagnosis, cure, mitigation, treatment, or prevention of disease or to affect the structure and function of the body.

Airlock

An enclosed space with two or more doors, which is interposed between two or more rooms, e.g. of differing classes of cleanliness, for the purpose of controlling the airflow between those rooms when they need to be entered. An airlock is designed for use either by people or for goods and/or equipment.

Authorized Person

The person recognized by the national regulatory authority as having the responsibility for ensuring that each batch of finished product has been manufactured, tested and approved for release in compliance with the laws and regulations in force in that country.

Batch (or lot)

A defined quantity of starting material, packing material, or product processed in a single process or series of processes so that it is expected to be homogeneous. It may sometimes be necessary to divide a batch into a number of sub-batches, which are later brought together to form a final homogeneous batch. In the case of terminal sterilization, the batch size is determined by the capacity of the autoclave. In continuous manufacture, the batch must correspond to a defined fraction of the production, characterized by its intended homogeneity. The batch size can be defined either as a fixed quantity or as the amount produced in a fixed time interval.

Batch Number (or lot number)

A distinctive combination of numbers and/or letters which uniquely identifies a batch on the labels, its batch records and corresponding certificates of analysis, etc.

Batch Records

All documents associated with the manufacture of a batch of bulk product or finished product. They provide a history of each batch of product and of all circumstances pertinent to the quality of the final product.

Bulk Product

Any product that has completed all processing stages up to, but not including, final packaging.

Calibration

The set of operations that establish, under specified conditions, the relationship between values indicated by an instrument or system for measuring, recording and controlling, or the values represented by a material measure, and the corresponding known values of a reference standard. Limits for acceptance of the results of measuring should be established.

Clean Area

An area with defined environmental control of particulate and microbial contamination, constructed and used in such a way as to reduce the introduction, generation, and retention of contaminants within the area.

Consignment (or Delivery)

The quantity of a pharmaceutical material(s), made by one manufacturer and supplied at one time in response to a particular request or order. A consignment may comprise one or more packages or containers and may include material belonging to more than one batch.

Contamination

The undesired introduction of impurities of a chemical or microbiological nature, or of foreign matter, into or on to a starting material or intermediate during production, sampling, packaging or repackaging, storage or transport.

Critical-Operation

An operation in the manufacturing process that may cause variation in the quality of the pharmaceutical product.

Cross-Contamination

Contamination of a starting material, intermediate product or finished product with another starting material or product during production.

Finished Product

A finished dosage form that has undergone all stages of manufacture, including packaging in its final container and labelling.

In-Process Control

Checks performed during production in order to monitor and, if necessary, to adjust the process to ensure that the product conforms to its specifications. The control of environment or equipment may also be regarded as a part of in-process control.

Intermediate Product

Partly processed product that must undergo further manufacturing steps before it becomes a bulk product.

Large-Volume Parenterals

Sterile solutions intended for parenteral application with a volume of 100mL or more in one container of the finished dosage form.

Manufacture

All operations of purchase of materials and products, production, quality control, release, storage and distribution of pharmaceutical products, and the related controls.

Manufacturer

A company that carries out operations such as production, packaging, repackaging, labelling and relabeling of pharmaceuticals.

Marketing Authorization (Product License, Registration Certificate)

A legal document issued by the competent drug regulatory authority that establishes the detailed composition and formulation of the product and the pharmacopoeial or other recognized specifications of its ingredients and of the final product itself, and includes details of packaging, labelling and shelf-life.

Master Formula

A document or set of documents specifying the starting materials with their quantities and the packaging materials, together with a description of the procedures and precautions required to produce a specified quantity of a finished product as well as the processing instructions, including the in-process controls.

Master Record

A document or set of documents that serve as a basis for the batch documentation (blank batch record)

Packaging

All operations, including filling and labelling, that a bulk product has to undergo in order to become a finished product. Filling of a sterile product under aseptic conditions or a product intended to be terminally sterilized, would not normally be regarded as part of packaging.

Packaging Material

Any material, including printed material, employed in the packaging of a pharmaceutical, but excluding any outer packaging used for transportation or shipment. Packaging materials are referred to as primary or secondary according to whether or not they are intended to be in direct contact with the product.

Pharmaceutical Product

Any material or product intended for human or veterinary use presented in its finished dosage form or as a starting material for use in such a dosage form that is subject to control by pharmaceutical legislation in the exporting state and/or the importing state.

Production

All operations involved in the preparation of pharmaceutical product, from receipt of materials, through processing, packaging and repackaging, labelling and relabeling, to completion of finished product.

Qualification

Action of proving that any premises, systems and items of equipment work correctly and actually lead to the expected results. The meaning of the word "validation" is sometimes extended to incorporate the concept of qualification.

Quarantine

The status of starting or packaging materials, intermediates, or bulk or finished products isolated physically or by other effective means while a decision is awaited on their release, rejection or reprocessing.

Reconciliation

A comparison between the theoretical quantity and the actual quantity.

Recovery

The introduction of all or part of previous batches (or of redistilled solvents and similar products) of the required quality into another batch at a defined stage of manufacture. It includes the removal of impurities from waste to obtain a pure substance or the recovery of used materials for a separate use.

Reprocessing

Subjecting all or part of a batch or lot of an in-process drug, bulk process intermediate (final biological bulk intermediate) or bulk product of a single batch/lot to a previous step in the validated manufacturing process due to failure to meet predetermined specifications. Reprocessing procedures are foreseen as occasionally necessary for biological drugs and, in such cases, are validated and pre-approved as part of the marketing authorization.

Reworking

Subjecting an in-process or bulk process intermediate (final biological bulk intermediate) or final product of a single batch to an alternate manufacturing process due to failure to meet predetermined specifications. Reworking is an unexpected occurrence and is not pre-approved as part of the marketing authorization.

Self-contained Area

Premises which provide complete and total separation of all aspects of an operation, including personnel and equipment movement, with well established procedures, controls and monitoring. This includes physical barriers as well as separate air-handling systems, but does not necessarily imply two distinct and separate buildings.

Specification

A list of detailed requirements with which the products or materials used or obtained during manufacture have to conform. They serve as a basis for quality evaluation.

Standard Operating Procedures (Sop)

An authorized written procedure giving instructions for performing operations not necessarily specific to a given product or material (e.g. equipment operation, maintenance and cleaning; validation; cleaning of premises and environmental control; sampling and inspection). Certain SOP's may be used to supplement product-specific master and batch production documentation.

Starting Material

Any substance of a defined quality used in the production of a pharmaceutical product, but excluding packaging material.

Validation

Action of proving, in accordance with the principles of GMP, that any procedure, process, equipment, material, activity or system actually leads to the expected results.

Summary of GMP Guidelines

Good Manufacturing Practices for Pharmaceutical Products (GMP)

Good manufacturing practice is that part of quality assurance which ensures that products are consistently produced and controlled to the quality standards appropriate to their intended use and as required by the marketing authorization. GMP are aimed primarily at diminishing the risks inherent in any pharmaceutical production. Such risks are essentially of two types: cross-contamination (in particular of unexpected contaminants) and mix-ups (confusion) caused by, for example, false labels being put on containers. Under GMP:

(a) All manufacturing processes are clearly defined, systematically reviewed in the light of experience, and shown to be capable of consistently manufacturing pharmaceutical products of the required quality that comply with their specifications;

(b) Qualification and validation are performed;

(c) All necessary resources are provided, including:

  (i) Appropriately qualified and trained personnel;

  (ii) Adequate premises and space;

  (iii) Suitable equipment and services;

  (iv) Appropriate materials, containers and labels;

  (v) Approved procedures and instructions;

(vi) Suitable storage and transport

(vii) Adequate personnel, laboratories and equipment for in-process controls;

(d) Instructions and procedures are written in clear and unambiguous language, specifically applicable to the facilities provided;

(e) Operators are trained to carry out procedures correctly;

(f) Records are made (manually and/or by recording instruments) during manufacture to show that all the steps required by the defined procedures and instructions have in fact been taken and that the quantity and quality of the product are as expected; any significant deviations are fully recorded and investigated;

(g) Records covering manufacture and distribution, which enable the complete history of a batch to be traced, are retained in a comprehensible and accessible form;

(h) The proper storage and distribution of the products minimizes any risk to their quality;

(i) A system is available to recall any batch of product from sale or supply;

(j) Complaints about marketed products are examined, the causes of quality defects investigated, and appropriate measures taken in respect of the defective products to prevent recurrence.

Components of GMP

Personnel

General

The establishment and maintenance of a satisfactory system of quality assurance and the correct manufacture and control of pharmaceutical products and active ingredients rely upon people. For this reason there must be sufficient qualified personnel to carry out all the tasks for which the manufacturer is responsible. Individual responsibilities should be clearly defined and understood by the persons concerned and recorded as written descriptions. The manufacturer should have an adequate number of personnel with the necessary qualifications and practical experience. The responsibilities placed on any one individual should not be so extensive so as to present any risk to quality. All responsible staff should have their specific duties recorded in written descriptions and adequate authority to carry out their responsibilities. Their duties may be delegated to designated deputies of a satisfactory qualification level. There should be no gaps or unexplained overlaps in the responsibilities of personnel concerned with the application of GMP. The manufacturer should have an organization chart.

All personnel should be aware of the principles of GMP that affect them and receive initial and continuing training, including hygiene instructions, relevant to their needs. All personnel should be motivated to support the establishment and maintenance of high-quality standards. Steps should be taken to prevent unauthorized people from entering production, storage and quality control areas. Personnel who do not work in these areas should not use them as passageway.

Key Personnel

Key personnel include the head of production, the head of quality control and the authorized person. Normally key posts should be occupied by full-time personnel. The heads of production and quality control should be independent of each other. In large organizations, it may be necessary to delegate some of the functions; however, the responsibility cannot be delegated. Key personnel responsible for supervising the manufacturing and quality control of pharmaceutical products should possess the qualifications of a scientific education and practical experience required by national legislation. Their education should include the study of an appropriate combination of:

(a) Chemistry or biochemistry
(b) Chemical engineering
(c) Microbiology
(d) Pharmaceutical sciences and technology
(e) Pharmacology and toxicology
(f) Physiology
(g) Other related sciences

They should also have adequate practical experience in the manufacture and quality assurance of pharmaceutical products. In order to gain such experience, a preparatory period may be required, during which they should exercise their duties under professional guidance. The scientific education and practical experience of experts should be such as to enable them to exercise independent professional judgement, based on the application of scientific principles and understanding to the practical problems encountered in the manufacture and quality control of pharmaceutical products.

The heads of the production and quality control generally have some shared, or jointly exercised, responsibilities relating to quality. These may include, depending on national regulations:

(a) Authorization of written procedures and other documents, including amendments;

(b) Monitoring and control of the manufacturing environment;
(c) Plant hygiene;
(d) Process validation and calibration of analytical apparatus;
(e) Training, including the application and principles of quality assurance;
(f) Approval and monitoring of suppliers of materials;
(g) Approval and monitoring of contract manufacturers;
(h) Designation and monitoring of storage conditions for materials and products;
(i) Performance and evaluation of in-process controls;
(j) Retention of records;
(k) Monitoring of compliance with GMP requirements;
(l) Inspection, investigation and taking of samples in order to monitor factors that may affect product quality.

Responsibilities of Head of Production

The head of the production generally has the following responsibilities:

(a) To ensure that products are produced and stored according to the appropriate documentation in order to obtain the required quality;
(b) To approve the instructions relating to production operations, including the in-process controls, and to ensure their strict implementation;
(c) To ensure that the production records are evaluated and signed by a designated person;
(d) To check the maintenance of the department, premises, and equipment;
(e) To ensure that the appropriate process validations and calibrations of control equipment are performed and recorded and the reports made available;
(f) To ensure that the required initial and continuing training of production personnel is carried out and adapted according to need.

Responsibilities of Head of Quality Control

The head of the quality control generally has the following responsibilities:

(a) To approve or reject starting materials, packaging materials, and intermediate, bulk and finished products in relation to their specifications;
(b) To evaluate batch records;

(c) To ensure that all necessary testing is carried out;
(d) To approve sampling instructions, specifications, test methods and other quality control procedures ;
(e) To approve and monitor analyses carried out under contract;
(f) To check the maintenance of the department, premises and equipment;
(g) To ensure that the appropriate validations, including those of analytical procedures, and calibrations of control equipment are carried out;
(h) To ensure that the required initial and continuing training of quality control personnel is carried out and adapted according to need.

The authorized person is responsible for compliance with technical or regulatory requirements related to the quality of finished products and the approval of the release of the finished product for sale.

The authorized person will also be involved in other activities, including the following:

(a) Implementation (and, when needed, establishment) of the quality system;
(b) Participation in the development of the company's quality manual;
(c) Supervision of the regular internal audits or self-inspections;
(d) Oversight of the quality control department;
(e) Participation in external audit (vendor audit);
(f) Participation in validation programmes.

The function of the approval of the release of a finished batch or a product can be delegated to a designated person with appropriate qualifications and experience who will release the product in accordance with an approved by means of batch review.

The person responsible for approving a batch for release should always ensure that the following requirements have been met:

(a) The marketing authorization and the manufacturing authorization requirements for the products have been met for the batch concerned;
(b) The principles and guidelines of GMP, as laid down in the guidelines published by WHO, have been followed;
(c) The principal manufacturing and testing processes have been validated, if different;

(d) All the necessary checks and tests have been performed and account taken of the production conditions and manufacturing records;

(e) Any planned changes or deviations in manufacturing or quality control have been notified in accordance with a well defined reporting system before any product id released. Such changes may need notification to, and approval by, the drug regulatory authority;

(f) Any additional sampling, inspection, tests and checks have been carried out or initiated, as appropriate, to cover planned changes and deviations;

(g) All necessary production and quality control documentation has been completed and endorsed by supervisors trained in appropriate disciplines;

(h) Appropriate audits, self-inspections and spot-checks are carried out by experienced and trained staff;

(i) Approval has been given by the head of quality control;

(j) All relevant factors have been considered, including any not specifically associated with the output batch directly under review (e.g. subdivision of output batches from a common input, factors associated with continuous production runs).

Training

The manufacturer should provide training in accordance with a written programme for all personnel whose duties take them into manufacturing areas or into control laboratories (including the technical, maintenance and cleaning personnel) and for other personnel required. Besides basic training on the theory and practice of GMP, newly recruited personnel should receive training appropriate to the duties assigned to them. Continuing training should also be given, and its practical effectiveness periodically assessed. Approved training programmes should be available. Training records should be kept. Personnel working in areas where contamination is a hazard, e.g. clean areas or areas where highly active, toxic, infectious or sensitizing materials are handled, should be given specific training. The concept of quality assurance and all the measures which aid its understanding and implementation should be fully discussed during the training sessions. Visitors or untrained personnel should preferably not be taken into the production and quality control areas. If this is unavoidable, they should be given relevant information in advance (particularly about personal hygiene) and the prescribed protective clothing. They should be closely supervised. Consultant and contract staff should be qualified for the services they provide. Evidence of this should be included in the training records.

Personal Hygiene

All personnel, prior to and during employment, as appropriate, should undergo health examinations. Personnel conducting visual inspections should also undergo periodic eye examinations. All personnel should be trained in the practices of personal hygiene. A high level of personal hygiene should be observed by all those concerned with manufacturing processes. In particular, personnel should be instructed to wash their hands before entering production areas. Signs to this effect should be posted and instructions observed. Any person shown at any time to have an apparent illness or open lesions that may adversely affect the quality of products should not be allowed to handle starting materials, packaging materials, in-process materials or drug products until the conditions no longer judged to be a risk. All employees should be instructed and encouraged to report to their immediate supervisor any conditions (relating to plant, equipment or personnel) that they consider may adversely affect the products. Direct contact should be avoided between the operator's hands and starting materials, primary packaging materials and intermediate or bulk product. To ensure protection of the product from contamination, personnel should wear clean body coverings appropriate to the duties they perform, including appropriate hair covering. Used clothes, if reusable, should be stored in separate closed containers until properly laundered and, if necessary, disinfected or sterilized. smoking, eating, drinking, chewing, and keeping plants, food, drink, smoking material and personal medicines should not be permitted in production, laboratory and storage areas, or in any other areas where they might adversely influence product quality. Personal hygiene procedures including the use of protective clothing should apply to all persons entering production areas, whether they are temporary or full-time employees or non-employees, e.g. contractors employees, visitors, senior managers and inspectors.

Premises

Premises must be located, designed, constructed, adapted, and maintained to suit the operations to be carried out.

General

The layout and design of premises must aim to minimize the risk of errors and permit effective cleaning and maintenance in order to avoid cross-contamination, build-up of dust or dirt, and, in general, any adverse effect on the quality of products. Where dust is generated (e.g. during sampling, weighing, mixing and processing operations, packaging of powder), measures should be taken to avoid cross-contamination and facilitate cleaning. Premises should be situated in an environment that, when considered together with measures to protect the manufacturing process, presents minimum risk of causing any contamination of materials or products. Premises used for the manufacture of finished products should be ensured that repair and maintenance operations do not present any hazard to the quality of products. Premises should be carefully maintained, and it should be ensured that repair and maintenance operations do not present any hazard to the quality of products. Premises should be cleaned and, where applicable, disinfected according to detailed written procedures. Records should be maintained. Electrical supply, lighting, temperature, humidity and ventilation should be appropriate and such that they do not adversely affect, directly or indirectly, either the pharmaceutical products during their manufacture and storage, or the accurate functioning of equipment. should be designed and equipped so as to afford maximum protection against the entry of insects, birds or other animals. There should be a procedure for rodent and pest control. Premises should be designed to ensure the logical flow of materials and personnel.

Ancillary Areas

Rest and refreshment rooms should be separate from manufacturing and control areas. Facilities for changing and storing clothes and for washing and toilet purposes should be easily accessible and appropriate for the number of users. Toilets should not communicate directly with production or storage areas. Maintenance workshops should if possible be separated from production areas. Whenever part and tools are stored in the production area, they should be kept in rooms or lockers reserved for that use. Animal houses should be well isolated from other areas, with separate entrance (animal access) and air-handling facilities.

Storage Areas

Storage areas should be of sufficient capacity to allow orderly storage of the various categories of materials and products with proper separation and segregation: starting and packaging materials, intermediates, bulk and finished products, products in quarantine, and released, rejected, returned or recalled products. storage areas should be designed or adapted to ensure good storage conditions. In particular, they should be clean, dry, sufficiently lit and maintained within acceptable temperature limits. Where special storage conditions are required (e.g. temperature, humidity) these should be provided, controlled, monitored and recorded where appropriate. Receiving and dispatch bays should be separated and protect materials and products from the weather. Receiving areas should be designed and equipped to allow containers of incoming materials to be cleaned if necessary before storage. Where quarantine status is ensured by storage in separate areas, these areas must be clearly marked and their access restricted to authorized personnel. Any system replacing the physical quarantine should give equivalent security. Segregation should be provided for the storage of rejected, recalled, or returned materials or products. Highly active and radioactive materials, narcotics, other dangerous drugs, and substances presenting special risks of abuse, fire or explosion should be stored in safe and secure areas. Printed packaging materials are considered critical to the conformity of the pharmaceutical product to its labelling and special attention should be paid to sampling and the safe and secure storage of these materials. There should normally be a separate sampling area for starting materials. (if sampling is performed in the storage area, it should be conducted in such a way as to prevent contamination or cross-contamination.)

Weighing Areas

The weighing of starting materials and the estimation of yield by weighing should be carried out in separate weighing areas designed for that use, for example with provisions for dust control. Such areas may be part of either storage or production areas.

Production Areas

In order to minimize the risk of a serious medical hazard due to cross-contamination, dedicated and self-contained facilities must be available for the production of particular pharmaceutical products, such as highly sensitizing materials (e.g. penicillin) or biological preparations (e.g. live microorganisms). The production of certain other highly active products, such as some antibiotics, hormones, cytotoxic substances and certain non-pharmaceutical products, should not be conducted in the same facilities. In exceptional cases, the principle of campaign working in the same facilities can be accepted provided that specific precautions are taken and the necessary validations (including cleaning validation) are made. The manufacture of technical poisons, such as pesticides and herbicides, should not be allowed in premises used for the manufacture of pharmaceutical products. Premises should preferably be laid out in such a way as to allow the production to take place in areas connected in a logical order corresponding to the sequence of the operations and to the requisite cleanliness levels. The adequacy of the working and in-process storage space should permit the orderly and logical positioning of equipment and materials so as to minimize the risk of confusion between different pharmaceutical products or their components, to avoid cross-contamination, and to minimize the risk of omission or wrong application of any of the manufacturing or control steps. Where starting and primary packaging materials and intermediate or bulk products are exposed to the environment, interior surfaces (walls, floors and ceilings) should be smooth and free from cracks and open joints, should not shed particulate matter, and should permit easy and effective cleaning and, if necessary, disinfection. Pipe work, light fittings, ventilation points and other services should be designed and sited to avoid the creation of recesses that are difficult to clean. As far as possible, for maintenance purposes, they should be accessible from outside the manufacturing areas. Drains should be of adequate size and designed and equipped to prevent back-flow. Open channels should be avoided where possible, but if they are necessary they should be shallow to facilitate cleaning and disinfection. Production areas should be effectively ventilated, with air-control facilities (including filtration of air to a sufficient level to prevent contamination and cross-contamination, as well as control of temperature and, where necessary, humidity) appropriate to the products handled, to the operations undertaken and to the eternal environment. These areas should be regularly monitored during both production and non-production periods to ensure compliance with their design specifications. Premises for the packaging of pharmaceutical products should be specifically designed and laid out so as to avoid mi-ups or cross-contamination. Production areas should be well lit, particularly where visual on-line controls are carried out.

Quality Control Areas

Quality control laboratories should be separated from production areas. Areas where biological, microbiological or radioisotope test methods are employed should be separated from each other. Quality control laboratories should be designed to suit the operations to be carried out in them. Sufficient space should be given to avoid mix-up's and cross-contamination. There should be adequate suitable storage space for samples, reference standards (if necessary, with cooling), solvents, reagents and records. The design of the laboratories should take into account the suitability of construction materials, prevention of fumes and ventilation. There should be separate air supply to laboratories and production areas. Separate air-handling units and other provisions are needed for biological, microbiological and radio isotope laboratories. A separate room may be needed for instruments to protect them against electrical interference, vibration, contact with excessive moisture and other eternal factors, or where it is necessary to isolate the instruments.

Sanitation and Hygiene

A high level of sanitation and hygiene should be practiced in every aspect of the manufacture of drug products. The scope of sanitation and hygiene covers personnel, premises, equipment and apparatus, production materials and containers, products for cleaning and disinfection, and anything that could become a source of contamination to the product. Potential sources of contamination should be eliminated through an integrated comprehensive programme of sanitation and hygiene.

CHPATER - 9

Good Manufacturing Practices (GMP)-Part II

(Equipment and Raw Materials)

Learning Objectives

To learn GMP Guidelines about:

- Equipment
- Materials
- Starting Materials
- Packing Materials
- Intermediate and Bulk Products
- Finished Products
- Rejected, Recovered, Reprocessed and Reworked Materials
- Recalled Products
- Returned Goods
- Regents and Culture Media
- Reference Standards
- Waste Materials

Guidelines for Equipment

Equipment must be located, designed, constructed, adapted, and maintained to suit the operations to be carried out. The layout and design of equipment must aim to minimize the risk of errors and permit effective cleaning and in general, any adverse effect on the quality of products. Equipment should be installed in such a way as to minimize any risk of error or of contamination. Fixed pipe work should be clearly labelled to indicate the contents and, where applicable, the direction of flow. All service piping's and devices should be adequately marked, and special attention paid to the provision of non-interchangeable connections or adaptors for dangerous gases and liquids. Balances and other measuring equipment of an appropriate range and precision should be available for production and control operations and should be calibrated on a scheduled basis. Production equipment should be thoroughly cleaned on a scheduled basis. Laboratory equipment and instruments should be suited to the testing procedures undertaken. Washing, cleaning and drying equipment should be chosen and used so as not to be a source of contamination. Production equipment should not present any hazard to the products. The parts of the production equipment that come into contact with the product must not be reactive, additive, or absorptive to an extent that would affect the quality of the product. Defective equipment should be removed from production and quality control areas. If this is not possible, it should be clearly labelled as defective to prevent use.Closed equipment should be used whenever appropriate. Where open equipment is used or equipment id opened, precautions should be taken to minimize contamination. Non-dedicated equipment should be cleaned according to validated cleaning procedures between production of different pharmaceutical products to prevent cross contamination. Current drawings of critical equipment and support systems should be maintained.

Materials

The main objective of a pharmaceutical plant is to produce finished products for patients use from a combination of materials (starting and packaging). Materials include starting materials, packaging materials, gases, solvents, process aids, reagents and labelling materials.

General

No materials used for operations such as cleaning, lubrication of equipment and pest control, should come into direct contact with the product. Where possible, such materials should be of a suitable grade (e.g. food grade) to minimize health risks. All incoming materials and finished products should be quarantined immediately after receipt or processing, until they are released for use or distribution. All materials and products should be stored under the appropriate conditions established by the manufacturer and in an orderly fashion to permit batch segregation and stock rotation by a first-expire, first-out rule. Water used in the manufacture of pharmaceutical products should be suitable for its intended use.

Starting Materials

The purchase of starting materials is an important operation that should involve staff who have a particular and thorough knowledge of the products and suppliers. Starting materials should be purchased only from approved suppliers and, where possible, directly from the producer. It also recommended that the specifications established by the manufacturer for the starting materials be discussed with the suppliers. It is of benefit that all critical aspects of the production and control of the starting material in question, including handling, labelling and packaging requirements as well as complaints and rejection procedures, are contractually agreed between the manufacturer and the supplier. For each consignment, the containers should be checked for at least integrity of package and the seal and for correspondence between the order, the delivery note, and the supplier's label. All incoming materials should be checked to ensure that the consignment corresponds to the order. Containers should be cleaned where necessary and labelled, if required, with the prescribed information. Where additional labels are attached to containers, the original information should not be lost. Damage to containers and any other problem that might adversely affect the quality of a material should be recorded and reported to the quality control department and investigated. If one delivery of material is made up of different batches, each batch must be considered as separate for sampling, testing and release. Starting materials in the storage area should be appropriately labelled. Labels should bear at least the following information:

(a) The designated name of the product and the internal code reference where applicable;

(b) The batch number given by the supplier and, on receipt, the control or batch number given by the manufacturer, if any, documented so as to ensure traceability;

(c) The status of the contents (e.g. on quarantine, on test, released, rejected, returned, recalled);

(d) Where appropriate, an expiry date or a date beyond which resting is necessary.

When fully validated computerized storage systems are used, not all of the above information need be in a legible form on the label.

There should be appropriate procedures or measures to ensure the identity of the contents of each container of starting material. Bulk containers from which samples have been drawn should be identified. Only starting materials released by the quality control department and within their shelf-life should be used. Starting materials should be dispensed only by designated persons, following a written procedure, to ensure that the correct materials are accurately weighed or measured into clean and properly labelled containers. Each dispensed material and its weight or volume should be independently checked and the check recorded. Materials dispensed for each batch of the final product should be kept together and conspicuously labelled as such.

Packing Materials

The purchase, handling and control of primary and printed packaging materials should be as for starting materials. Particular attention should be paid to printed packaging materials. They should be stored in secure conditions so as to exclude the possibility of unauthorized access. Roll-feed labels should be used whenever possible. Cut labels and other loose printed materials should be stored and transported in separate closed containers so as to avoid mix-up. Packaging material should be issued for use only by designated personnel following an approved documented procedure. Each delivery or batch of printed or primary packaging material should be given a specific reference number or identification mark. Out dated or obsolete primary packaging material or printed packaging material should be destroyed and its disposal recorded. All products and packaging materials to be used should be checked on delivery to the packaging department for quantity, identify and conformity with the packaging instructions.

Intermediate and Bulk Products

Intermediate and bulk products should be kept under appropriate conditions. Intermediate and bulk products purchased as such should be handled on receipt as though they were starting materials.

Finished Products

Finished products should be held in quarantine until their final release, after which they should be stored as usable stock under conditions established by the manufacturer. The evaluation of finished products and the documentation necessary for release of a product for sale are described in section 17, "Good practices in quality control".

Rejected, Recovered, Reprocessed and Reworked Materials

Rejected materials and products should be clearly marked as such and stored separately in restricted areas. They should either be returned to the suppliers or, where appropriate, reprocessed or destroyed in a timely manner. Whatever action is taken should be approved by authorized personnel and recorded. The reworking or recovery of rejected products should be exceptional. It is permitted only if the quality of the final product is not affected, if the specifications are met, and if it is done in accordance with a defined and authorized procedure after evaluation of the risks involved. A record should be kept of the reworking or recovery. A reworked batch should be given a new batch number. The introduction of all or part earlier batches, conforming to the required quality, into a batch of the same product at a defined stage of manufacture should be authorized beforehand. This recovery should be carried out in according with a defined procedure after evaluation of the risks involved, including any possible effect on shelf-life. The recovery should be recorded. The need for additional testing of any finished product that has been reprocessed, reworked or into which a recovered product has been incorporated, should be considered by the quality control department.

Recalled Products

Recalled products should be identified and stored separately in a secure area until a decision is taken on their fate. The decision should be made as soon as possible.

Returned Goods

Products returned from the market should be destroyed unless it is certain that their quality is satisfactory; in such cases they may be considered for release or relabeling, or alternative action taken only after they have been critically assessed by the quality control function in accordance with a written procedure. The nature of the product, any special storage conditions it requires, its conditions and history, and the time elapsed since it was issued should all be taken into account in this assessment. Where any doubt arises over the quality of the product, it should not be considered suitable for reissue or reuse. Any action taken should be appropriately recorded.

Reagents and Culture Media

There should be records for the receipt and preparation of reagents and culture media. Reagents made up in the laboratory should be prepared according to written procedures and appropriately labelled. The label should indicate the concentration, standardisation factor, shelf-life, the date when restandardization is due, and the storage conditions. The label should be signed and dated by the person preparing the reagent. Both positive and negative controls should be applied to verify the suitability of culture media each time they are prepared and used. The size of the inoculum used in positive controls should be appropriate to the sensitivity required.

Reference Standards

Whenever official reference standards exist, there should preferably be used. Official reference standards should be used only for the purpose described in the appropriate monograph. Reference standards prepared by the producer should be tested, released and stored in the same way as official standards. They should be kept under the responsibility of a designated person in a secure area. Secondary or working standards may be established by the application of appropriate tests and checks at regular intervals to ensure standardization. Reference standards should be properly labelled with at least the following information:

(a) Name of material;

(b) Batch or lot number and control number;

(c) Date of preparation;

(d) Shelf-life;

(e) Potency;

(f) Storage conditions;

Waste Materials

Provision should be made for the proper and safe storage of waste materials awaiting disposal. Toxic substances and flammable materials should be stored in suitably designed, separate, enclosed cupboards, as required by national legislation. Waste materials should not be allowed to accumulate. It should be collected in suitable receptacles for removal to collection points outside the buildings and disposed of safely and in a sanitary manner at regular and frequent intervals.

Miscellaneous

Rodenticides, insecticides, fuming agents and sanitizing materials should not be permitted to contaminate equipment, starting materials, packaging materials, in-process materials or finished products.

CHPATER - 10

Good Manufacturing Practices (GMP) - Part III

(Documentation and Records)

Learning Objectives

To learn GMP Guidelines about

- Documentation
- General
- Documents Required
  - Labels,
  - Specifications and Testing Procedures,
  - Specifications for Starting and Packaging Materials,
  - Specifications for Intermediate and Bulk Products,
  - Specifications for Finished Products.
- Master Formulae
- Packaging Instructions
- Batch Processing Records
- Batch Packaging Records
- Standard Operating Procedures (SOPs)
- Records

Documentation

Good documentation is an essential part of the quality assurance system and, as such, should exist for all aspects of GMP. Its aims are to be define the specifications and procedures for all materials and methods of manufacture and control; to ensure that all personnel concerned with manufacture know what to do and when to do it; to ensure that authorized persons have all the information necessary to decide whether or not to release a batch of a drug for sale, to ensure the existence of documented evidence, traceability, and to provide records and an audit trail that will permit investigation. It ensures the availability of the data needed for validation, review and statistical analysis. The design and use of documents depend upon manufacturer. In some cases some or all of the documents described below may be brought together, but they will usually be separate.

General

Documents should be designed, prepared, reviewed and distributed with care. They should comply with the relevant parts of the manufacturing and marketing authorization. Documents should be approved, signed and dated by the appropriate responsible persons. No document should be changed without authorization and approval. Documents should have unambiguous contents: the title, nature and purpose should be clearly stated. They should be laid out in an orderly fashion and be easy to check. Reproduced documents should be clear and legible. The reproduction of working documents from master documents should be retained for a specific period of time. Documents should be regularly reviewed and kept up to date. When a document has been revised, a system should exist to prevent inadvertent use of the superseded version. Superseded documents should be retained for a specific period of time. Where documents require the entry of data, these entries should be clear, legible and indelible. Sufficient space should be provided for such entries. Any alteration made to a document should be signed and dated; the alteration should permit the reading of the original information. Where appropriate the reason for the alteration should be recorded. Records should be made or completed when any action is taken and in such a way that all significant activities concerning the manufacture of pharmaceutical products are traceable. Records should be retained for at least one year after the expiry date of finished product. Data (and records for storage) may be recorded by electronic data-processing systems or by photographic or other reliable means. Master formulae and detailed standard operating procedures relating to the system in use should be checked. If documentation is handled by electronic data-processing methods, only authorized persons should be able to enter or modify data in the computer, and there should be a record of changes and deletions; access should be restricted by passwords or other means and the entry of critical data should be independently checked. Batch records stored electronically should be protected by back-up transfer on magnetic tape, microfilm, paper print-outs or other names. It is particularly important that, during the period of retention, the data are readily available.

Documents Required

Labels

Labels applied to containers, equipment or premises should be clear, unambiguous and in the company's agreed format. It is often helpful in addition to the wording on the labels to use colours to indicate status (e.g. quarantined, accepted, rejected, and clean).

All finished drug products should be identified by labelling, as required by the national legislation, bearing at least the following information:

(a) The name of the drug product;
(b) A list of the active ingredients (if applicable, with the INNs) showing the amount of each present and a statement of the net contents (e.g. number of dosage units, weight, volume);
(c) The batch number assigned by the manufacturer;
(d) The expiry date in an uncoded form;
(e) Any special storage conditions or handling preparations that may be necessary;
(f) Directions for use, and warnings and precautions that may be necessary;
(g) The name and address of the manufacturer or the company or the person responsible for placing the product on the market.

For reference standards, the label and/or accompanying document should indicate potency or concentration, date of manufacture, expiry date, date the closure is first opened, storage conditions and control number, as appropriate.

Specifications and Testing Procedures

Testing procedures described in documentation should be validated in the context of available facilities and equipment before they are adapted for routine. There should be appropriately authorized and dated specifications, including tests on identity, content, purity and quality, for starting and packaging materials and for finished products; where appropriate, they should also be available for intermediate or bulk products. Specifications for water, solvents and reagents (e.g. acids and bases) used in production should be included. Each specification should be approved, signed and dated, and maintained by quality control, quality assurance unit or documentation centre. Periodic revisions of the specifications may be necessary to comply with new editions of the national pharmacopoeia or other official compendia. Pharmacopoeias, reference standards, reference spectra and other reference materials should be available in the quality control laboratory.

Specifications for Starting and Packaging Materials

Specifications for starting, primary and printed packaging materials should provide, if applicable, a description of the materials, including:

(a) The designed name and the internal code reference
(b) The reference, if any, to a pharmacopoeial monograph
(c) Qualitative and quantitative requirements with acceptance limits

Depending on the company's practice other data may be added to the specification, such as:

(a) The supplier and the original producer of the materials;
(b) A specimen of printed materials;
(c) Directions for sampling and testing, or a reference to procedures;
(d) Storage conditions and precautions;
(e) The maximum period of storage before re-examination.

Packaging material should conform to specifications, and should be compatible with the material and/or with the drug product it contains. The material should be examined for compliance with the specification, and for defects as well as for the correctness of identity markings. Documents describing testing procedures should state the required frequency for re-assaying each starting material, as determined by its stability.

Specifications for Intermediate and Bulk Products

Specifications for intermediate and bulk products should be available. The specifications should be similar to specifications for starting materials or for finished products, as appropriate.

Specifications for Finished Products

Specifications for finished products should include:

(a) The designed name of the product and the code reference, where applicable;
(b) The designed name(s) of the active ingredients(s) (if applicable, with the INNs);
(c) The formula or a reference to the formula;
(d) A description of the dosage form and package details;
(e) Direction of sampling and testing or a reference to procedures;
(f) The qualitative and quantitative requirements, with acceptable limits;
(g) The storage conditions and precautions, where applicable;
(h) The shelf-life.

Master Formulae

A formally authorized master formula should exist for each product and batch size to be manufactured.

The master formula should include:

(a) The name of the product, with a product reference code relating to its specification;
(b) A description of the dosage form, strength of the product and batch size;
(c) A list of all starting materials to be used (if applicable with the INNs), with the amount of each, described using the designated name and reference that is unique to that material (mention should be made of any substance that may disappear in the course of processing);
(d) A statement of the expected final yield with the acceptable limits, and of relevant intermediate yields, where applicable;
(e) A statement of the processing location and the principal equipment to be used;
(f) The methods, or reference to the methods, to be used for preparing and operating the critical equipment, e.g. cleaning (especially after a change in product), assembling, calibrating, sterilizing, use;
(g) Detailed step-wise processing instructions (e.g. checks on materials, pre-treatments, sequence for adding materials, mixing times, temperatures);
(h) The instructions for any in-processes controls with their materials
(i) Where necessary, the requirements for storage of the products, including the container, the labelling, and any special storage conditions;
(j) Any special precautions to be observed.

Packaging Instructions

Formally authorized packaging instructions should exist for each product, pack size and type. These should normally include, or make reference to:

(a) The name of the product;
(b) A description of its pharmaceutical form, strength and, where applicable, method of application;
(c) The pack size expressed in terms of the number, weight or volume of the product in the final container;
(d) A complete list of all the packaging materials required for a standard batch size, including quantities, sizes and types, with the code or

reference number relating to the specifications for each packaging material;

(e) Where appropriate, an example or reproduction of the relevant printed packaging materials and specimens, indicating where the batch number and expiry date of the product have been marked.

(f) Special precautions to be observed, including a careful examination of the packaging area and equipment in order to ascertain the line clearance before and after packaging operations.

(g) A description of the packaging operation, including any significant subsidiary operations, and equipment to be used;

(h) Details of in-process controls with instructions for sampling and acceptance limits.

Batch Processing Records

A batch processing record should be kept for each batch processed. It should be based on the relevant parts of the currently approved specifications on the record. The method of preparation of such records should be designed to avoid errors. (Copying or validated computer programmes are recommended. Transcribing from approved documents should be avoided). Before any processing begins, a check should be made that the equipment and workstation are clear of previous products, documents, or materials not required for the planned process, and that the equipment is clean and suitable for use. This check should be recorded. During processing, the following information should be recorded at the time each action is taken, and after completion the record should be dated and signed by the person responsible for the processing operations:

(a) The name of the product;

(b) The number of the batch being manufactured;

(c) Dates and times of commencement, of significant immediate stages, and of completion of production;

(d) The name of the person responsible for each stage of production;

(e) The initials of the operator(s) of different significant steps of production and, where appropriate, of the person(s) who checked each of these operations (e.g. weighing);

(f) The batch number and/or analytical control number and the quantity of each starting material actually weighed (including the batch number and amount of any recovered or reprocessed material added);

(g) Any relevant processing operation or event and the major equipment used;

(h) Then in-process controls performed, the initials of the person(s) carrying them out, and the results obtained;

(i) The amount of product obtained at different and pertinent stages of manufacture (yield), together with comments or explanations for significant deviations from the expected yield;

(j) Notes on special problems including details, with signed authorization for any deviation from the master formula;

Batch Packaging Records

A batch packaging record should be kept for each batch or part batch processed. It should be based on the relevant parts of the approved packaging instructions, and the method of preparing such records should be designed to avoid errors. (copying or validated computer programmes are recommended. Transcribing from approved documents should be avoided. Before any packaging operation begins, checks should be made that the equipment and work station are clear of previous products, documents or materials are not required for the planned packaging operations, and that equipment is clean and suitable for use. These checks should be recorded.

The following information should be recorded at that time each action is taken, and the date and the person responsible should be clearly identified by signature or electronic password:

(a) The name of the product, the batch number and the quantity of the bulk product to be packed, as well as the batch number and the planned quantity of finished product that will be obtained, the quantity actually obtained and the reconciliation;

(b) The date(s) and time(s) of the packaging operations;

(c) The name of the responsible person carrying out the packaging operation;

(d) The initials of the operators of the different significant steps;

(e) The checks made for identity and conformity with the packaging instructions, including the results of in-process controls;

(f) Details of the packaging operations carried out, including references to equipment and the packaging lines used, and when necessary, the instructions for keeping the product unpacked or a record of returning product that has been packaged to the storage area;

(g) Whenever possible, samples of the printed packaging materials used, including specimens bearing the approval for the printing of and regular check (where appropriate) of the batch number, expiry date, and any additional overprinting

(h) The quantities and reference number or identification of all printed packaging materials and bulk product issued, used, destroyed or returned to stock and the quantities of product obtained to permit an adequate reconciliation.

Standard Operating Procedures (SOPs) Records

Standard operating procedures and associated records of actions taken or, where appropriate, conclusions reached should be available for:

(a) Equipment assembly and validation;
(b) Analytical apparatus and calibration;
(c) Maintenance, cleaning and sanitization;
(d) Personnel matters including qualification, training, clothing and hygiene;
(e) Environmental monitoring;
(f) Pest control;
(g) Complaints;
(h) Recalls;
(i) Returns;

There should be standard operating procedures and records for the receipt of each delivery of starting material and primary and printed packaging material.

The records of the receipts should include:

(a) The name of the material on the delivery note and the containers;
(b) The "in-house" name and/or code of material if different from (a);
(c) The date of receipt;
(d) The supplier's name and, if possible, manufacturers name;
(e) The manufacturer's batch or reference number;
(f) The total quantity, and number of containers received;
(g) The batch number assigned after receipt;
(h) Any relevant comment (e.g. state of the containers).

There should be standard operating procedures for the internal labelling, quarantine and storage of starting materials, packaging materials and other materials as appropriate. Standard operating procedures should be available for each instrument and piece of equipment (e.g. use, calibration, cleaning, maintenance) and placed in close proximity to the equipment. There should be standard operating procedures for sampling, which specify the person(s) authorized to take samples.

The sampling instructions should include:

(a) The method of sampling and the sampling plan;
(b) The equipment to be used;

(c) Any precautions to be observed to avoid contamination of the material or any deterioration in its quality;
(d) The amount of samples to be taken
(e) Instruction for any required subdivision of the sample;
(f) The type of sample container to be used and whether they are for aseptic sampling or for normal sampling, and labelling;
(g) Any specific precautions to be observed, especially in regard to the sampling of sterile or noxious material.

There should be a standard operating procedure describing the details of the batch (lot) numbering system, with the objective of ensuring that each batch of intermediate, bulk or finished product is identified with a specific batch number. The standard operating procedures for batch numbering that are applied to the processing stage and to the respective packaging stage should be related to each other. The standard operating procedures for batch numbering should ensure that the same batch numbers will not be used repeatedly; this applies also to reprocessing. Batch-number allocation should be immediately recorded, e.g. in a log-book. The record should include at least the date of collection, product identity and size of batch. There should be written procedures for testing materials and products at different stages of manufacture, describing the methods and equipment to be used. The tests performed should be recorded.

Analysis records should include at least the following data:

(a) The name of the material or product and, where applicable, dosage form;
(b) The batch number and, where appropriate, the manufacturer and/or supplier;
(c) References to the relevant specifications and testing procedures;
(d) Test results, including observations and calculations, and reference to any specifications;
(e) Date and reference number of testing;
(f) The initials of the persons who performed the testing;
(g) The date and initials of the persons who verified the testing and the calculations, where appropriate;
(h) A clear statement of release or rejection and the dated signature of the designated responsible person.

Written release and rejection procedures should be available for materials and products, and in particular for the release for sale of the finished product by an authorized person. Records should be maintained of the distribution of each batch of a product in order. e.g. to facilitate the recall of the batch if necessary. Records should be kept for major and critical equipment, as appropriate, of any validations, calibrations, maintenance, cleaning, or repair operations, including dates and the identity of the people who carried these operations out. The use of major and critical equipment and the areas where products have been processed should be appropriately recorded in chronological order. There should be written procedures assigning responsibility for cleaning and sanitation and describing in sufficient detail the cleaning schedules, methods, equipment and materials to be used and facilities and equipment to be cleaned. Such written procedures should be followed.

CHPATER - 11

Good Manufacturing Practices (GMP) –Part IV

(Good Practices in Production and Quality Control, Quality Audits and Complains)

Learning Objectives

To learn GMP Guidelines about:

- Qualification and validation
- Good Practices in Production
- Prevention of Cross-Contamination and Bacterial Contamination during Production
- Processing Operations
- Packaging Operations
- Good Practices in Quality Control
- Control of Starting Materials and Intermediate, Bulk and Finished Products
- Test Requirements for
    - Starting and Packaging Materials
    - In process Control
    - Finished Products
- Batch Record Review
- Stability Studies
- Complaints
- Product Recalls
- Self Inspection and Quality Audits
- Self Inspection Report
- Quality Audit
- Suppliers Audits and Approval

Good Practices in Production

Principle. Production operations must follow clearly defined procedures in accordance with manufacturing and marketing authorizations, with the objective of obtaining products of the requisite quality.

General

All handling of materials and products, such as receipt and cleaning, quarantine, sampling, storage, labelling, dispensing, processing, packaging and distribution, should be done in accordance with written procedures or instructions and where necessary, recorded. Any deviation from instructions or procedures should be avoided as far as possible. If deviations occur, they should be in accordance with an approved procedure. The authorization of the deviation should be approved in writing by a designated person, with the involvement of the quality control department, when appropriate. Checks on yields and reconciliation of quantities should be carried out as necessary to ensure that there are no discrepancies outside acceptable limits. Operations on different products should not be carried out simultaneously or consecutively in the same room or area unless there is no risk of mix-up or cross-contamination. At all times during processing, all materials, bulk containers, major items of equipment, and where appropriate, the rooms and packaging lines being used should be labelled or otherwise identified with an indication of the product or material being processed, its strength and the batch number. Where applicable, this indication should also mention the stage of production. In some cases, it may be useful to record also the name of the previous product that has been processed. Access to production premises should be restricted to authorized personnel. Normally, non-medical products should not be restricted in areas or with equipment destined for the production of pharmaceutical products. In-process controls are usually performed within the production area. The performance of such in-process controls should not have any negative effect on the quality of the product or another product (e.g. cross-contamination or mix-up).

Prevention of Cross-Contamination and Bacterial Contamination during Production

When dry materials and products are used in production, special precaution should be taken to prevent the generation and dissemination of dust. Provision should be made for proper air control (e.g. supply and extraction of air of suitable quality). Contamination of a starting material or of a product by another material or product must be avoided. The risk of accidental cross-contamination arises from the uncontrolled release of dust, gases, particles, vapours, sprays or organisms from materials and products in process, from residues on equipment, from intruding insects, and from operators clothing, skin, etc. The significance of the risk varies with the type of contaminant and of the product being contaminated. Among the most hazardous contaminants are highly sensitizing materials, biological preparations such as living organisms, certain hormones, cytotoxic substances, and other highly active materials. Products in which contamination is likely to be most significant are those administered by injection or applied to open wounds and those given in large doses and/or over a long time. Cross-contamination should be avoided by taking appropriate technical or organizational measures, for example:

(a) Carrying out production in dedicated and self-contained areas (which may be required for products such as penicillin, live vaccines, live bacterial preparations and certain other biological);
(b) Conducting campaign production (separation in time) followed by appropriate cleaning in accordance with a validated cleaning procedure;
(c) Providing appropriately designed airlocks, pressure differentials, and air supply and extraction systems.
(d) Minimizing the risk of contamination caused by recirculation or re-entry of untreated or insufficiently treated air;
(e) Wearing protective clothing where products or materials are handled;
(f) Using cleaning and documentation procedures of known effectiveness;
(g) Using a closed system in production;
(h) Testing for residues;
(i) Using cleanliness status labels on equipment.

Measures to prevent cross-contamination and their effectiveness should be checked periodically according to standard operating procedures. Production areas where susceptible products are processed should undergo periodic environmental monitoring (e.g. for microbiological monitoring and particulate matter where appropriate).

Processing Operations

Before any processing operation is started, steps should be taken to ensure that the work area and equipment are clean and free from any starting materials, products, product residues, labels or documents not required for the current operation. Any necessary in-process controls and environmental controls should be carried out and recorded. Means should be instituted of indicating failures of equipment or of services (e.g. water, gas) to equipment. Defective equipment should be withdrawn from use until the defect has been rectified. After use, production equipment should be cleaned without delay according to detailed written procedures and stored under clean and dry conditions in a separate area or in a manner that will prevent contamination. Time limits for storage of equipment after cleaning and before use should be stated and based on data. Containers for filling should be cleaned before filling. Attention should be given to avoiding and removing any contaminants such as glass fragments and metal particles. Any significant deviation from the expected yield should be recorded and investigated. Checks should be carried out to ensure that pipelines and other pieces of equipment used for the transportation of products from one area to another and connected in a correct manner. Pipes used for conveying distilled or deionized water and, where appropriate, other water pipes should be sanitized and stored according to written procedures that detail the action limits for microbiological contamination and the measures to be taken. Measuring, weighing, recording, and control equipment and instruments should be serviced and calibrated at prespecified intervals and records maintained. To ensure satisfactory functioning, instruments should be checked daily or prior to use for performing analytical tests. The date of calibration and servicing and the date when recalibration is due should be clearly indicated, preferably on a label attached to the instrument. Repair and maintenance operations should not present any hazard to the quality of products.

Packaging Operations

When the programme for packaging operations is being set up, particular attention should be given to minimizing the risk of contamination, mix-ups or substitutions. Different products should not be packaged in close proximity unless there is physical segregation or an alternative system that will provide equal assurance. Before packaging operations are begun, steps should be taken to ensure that the work area, packaging lines, printing machines and other equipment are clean and free from any products, materials or documents used previously and which are not required for the current operation. The line clearance should be performed according to an appropriate procedures and check list and recorded. The name and batch number of the product being handled should be displayed at each packaging station or line. Normally, filling and sealing should be followed as quickly as possible by labelling. If labelling is delayed, appropriate procedures should be applied to ensure that no mix-ups or mislabeling can occur. The correct performance of any printing (e.g. of code numbers or expiry dates) done separately or in the course of the packaging should be checked and recorded. Attention should be paid to printing by hand, which should be rechecked at regular intervals. Special care should be taken when cut labels are used and when over-printing is carried out off-line, and in hand-packing operations. Roll-feed labels are normally preferable to cut labels in helping to avoid mix-ups. Online verification of all labels by automated electronic means can be helpful in preventing mix-ups, but checks should be made to ensure that any electronic code readers, label counters, or similar devices are operating correctly. When labels are attached manually, in-process control checks should be performed more frequently. Printed and embossed information on packaging materials should be distinct and resistant to fading or erasing. Regular on-line control of the product during packaging should include at least checks on:

(a) The general appearance of the packages;
(b) Whether the packages are complete;
(c) Whether the correct products and packaging materials are used;
(d) Whether any overprinting is correct;
(e) The correct functioning of line monitors.

Samples taken away from the packaging line should not be returned.

Products that have been involved in an unusual event during packaging should be reintroduced into the process only after special inspection, investigation and approval by authorized personnel. A detailed record should be kept of this operation. Any significant or unusual discrepancy observed during reconciliation of the amount of bulk product and printed packaging materials and the number of units produced should be investigated, satisfactorily accounted for, and recorded before release. Upon completion of a packaging operation, any unused batch-coded packaging materials should be destroyed, and the destruction recorded. A documented procedure requiring checks to be performed before returning unused materials should be followed if uncoded printed materials are returned to check.

Good Practices in Quality Control

Quality control is the part of GMP concerned with sampling, specifications and testing, and with the organization, documentation and release procedures which ensure that the necessary and relevant tests are actually carried out and that materials are not released for use, nor products released for sale or supply, until their quality has been judged to be satisfactory. Quality control is not confirmed to laboratory operations but must be involved in all decisions concerning the quality of the product. The independence of quality control from production is considered functional.

Each manufacturer (the holder of a manufacturing authorization) should have a quality control function. The quality control function should be independent of other departments and under the authority of a person with appropriate qualifications and experience, who has one or several control laboratories at his or her disposal. Adequate resources must be available to ensure that all the quality control arrangements are effectively and reliably carried out. The basic requirements for quality control are as follows:

(a) Adequate facilities, trained personnel and approved procedures must be available for sampling, inspecting, and testing starting materials, packaging materials, and intermediate, bulk, and finished products, and where appropriate for monitoring environmental conditions for GMP purposes;

(b) Samples of starting materials, packaging materials, intermediate products, bulk products and finished products must be taken by methods and personnel approved of by the quality control department;

(c) Qualification and validation must be performed;

(d) Records must be made demonstrating that all the required sampling. Inspecting and testing procedures have actually been carried out and that any deviations have been fully recorded and investigated;

(e) The finished products must contain ingredients complying with the qualitative and quantitative composition of the product described in the marketing authorization; the ingredients must be of the required purity, in their proper container and correctly labelled;

(f) Records must be made of the results of inspecting and testing the materials and intermediate, bulk and finished products against specifications; product assessment must include a review and evaluation of the relevant production documentation and an assessment of deviations from specified procedures;

(g) No batch of product is to be released for sale or supply prior to certification by the authorized person(s) that it is an accordance with the requirements of the marketing authorization. In certain countries, by law, the batch release is a task of the authorized person from production together with the authorized person from quality control;

(h) Sufficient samples of starting materials and products must be retained to permit future examination of the product if necessary; the retained product must be kept in its final pack unless the pack is exceptionally large.

Quality control as a whole will also have other duties, such as to establish, validate and implement all quality control procedures, to evaluate, maintain, and store the reference standards for substances, to ensure that the stability of the active pharmaceutical ingredients and products is monitored, to participate in the investigation of complaints related to the quality of the product, and to participate in the investigation of complaints related to the quality of the product, and to participate in environmental monitoring. All these operations should be carried out in accordance with written procedures and, where necessary, recorded.

Assessment of finished products should embrace all relevant factors, including the production of conditions, the results of in-process testing, manufacturing, documentation, compliance with the specification for the finished product, and an examination of the finished pack. Quality control personnel must have access to production areas of sampling and investigation as appropriate.

Control of Starting Materials and Intermediate, Bulk and Finished Products

All tests should follow the instructions given in the relevant written test procedure for each material or product. The result should be checked by the supervisor before the material or product is released or rejected. Samples should be representative of the batches of material from which they are taken in accordance with the approved written procedure. Sampling should be carried out so as to avoid contamination or other adverse effects on quality. The containers that have been sampled should be marked accordingly and carefully resealed after sampling. Care should be taken during sampling to guard against contamination or mix-up of, or by, the material being sampled. All sampling equipment that comes into contact with the material should be clean. Some particularly hazardous or potent materials may require special precautions. Sampling equipment should be cleaned and, if necessary, sterilized before and after each use and stored separately from other laboratory equipment.

Each sample container should bear a label indicating:

(a) The name of the sampled material;

(b) The batch or lot number;

(c) The number of the container from which the sample has taken;

(d) The number of the sample;

(e) The signature of the person who has taken the sample;

(f) The date of sampling.

Out-of-specification results obtained during testing of materials or products should be investigated in accordance with an approved procedure. Records should be maintained.

Test Requirements

Starting and Packaging Materials

Before releasing a starting or packaging material for use, the quality control manager should ensure that the materials have been tested for conformity with specifications for identity, strength, purity and other quality parameters. An identity test should be conducted on a sample from each container of starting material. Each batch of printed packaging materials must be examined following receipt. In lieu of testing by the manufacturer, a certificate of analysis may be accepted from the supplier, provided the manufacturer establishes the reliability of the supplier's analysis through appropriate periodic validation of the supplier's test results and through on-site audits of the supplier's capabilities. Certificates must be originals or otherwise have their authenticity assured. Certificates must contain at least the following information;

(a) Identification of the issuing supplier;
(b) Signature of the competent official and statement of his or her qualifications;
(c) The name of the material tested;
(d) The batch number of the material tested;
(e) The specifications and methods used;
(f) The test result obtained;
(g) The date of testing;

In-Process Control

In-process control records should be maintained and from a part of the batch records.

Finished Products

For each batch of the drug product, there should be an appropriate laboratory determination of satisfactory conformity to its finished product specification prior to release. Products failing to meet the established specifications or any other relevant quality criteria should be rejected.

Batch Record Review

Production and quality control records should be reviewed as part of the approval process of batch release. Any divergence or failure of a batch to meet its specifications should be thoroughly investigated. The investigation should, if necessary, extend to other batches of the same product and other products that may have been associated with the specific failure or discrepancy. A written record of the investigation should be made and should include the conclusion and follow-up action. Retention samples from each batch of finished product should be kept for at least one year after the expiry date. Finished products should usually be kept in their final packaging and stored under the recommended conditions. If exceptionally large packages are produced, smaller samples might be stored in appropriate containers. Samples of active starting materials should be retained for at least one year beyond the expiry date of the corresponding finished product. Other starting materials should be retained for a minimum for 2 years if their stability allows. Retention samples of materials and products should be of a size sufficient to permit at least two full re-examinations.

Stability Studies

Quality control should evaluate the quality and stability of finished pharmaceutical products and, when necessary, of starting materials and intermediate products. Quality control should establish expiry dates and shelf-life specifications on the basis of stability tests related to storage conditions. A written programme for on-going stability determination should be developed and implemented to include elements such as:

(a) A complete description of the drug involved in the study;

(b) The complete set of testing parameters and methods, describing all tests for potency, purity, and physical characteristics and documented evidence that these tests indicate stability;

(c) Provision for special storage conditions;

(d) Provision for the inclusion of a sufficient number of batches;

(e) The testing schedule for each drug;

(f) Provision for adequate sample retention;

(g) A summary of all the data generated, including the evaluation and the conclusions of the study. Stability should be determined prior to marketing and following any significant changes in processes, equipment, packaging materials, etc.

Complaints

All complaints and other information concerning potentially defective products should be carefully reviewed according to written procedures and the corrective action should be taken. A person responsible for handling the complaints and deciding the measures to be taken should be designated, together with sufficient supporting staff to assist him or her. If this person is different from the authorized person, the latter should be made aware of any complaint, investigation or recall. There should be written procedures describing the action to be taken, including the need to consider a recall, in the case of complaint concerning a possible product defect. Special attention should be given to establishing whether a complaint was caused because of counterfeiting. Any complaint concerning a product defect should be recorded with all the original details and thoroughly investigated. The person responsible for quality control should be normally be involved in the review of such investigations. If a product defect is discovered or suspected in a batch, consideration should be given to whether other batches should be checked in order to determine whether they also affected. In particular, other batches that may contain reprocessed product from the defective batch should be investigated. Where necessary, appropriate follow-up action, possibly including product recall, should be taken after investigation and evaluation of the complaint. All decisions made and measures taken as a result of complaint should be recorded and referenced to the corresponding batch records. Complaints records should be regularly reviewed for any indication of specific or recurring problems that require attention and might justify the recall of marketed products. The competent authorities should be informed if a manufacturer is considering action following possibly faculty manufacture, product deterioration, counterfeiting or any other serious quality problems with a product.

Product Recalls

There should be a system to recall from the market, promptly and effectively, products known or suspected to be defective. The authorized person should be responsible for the execution and coordination of recalls. He/she should have sufficient staff to handle all aspects of the recalls with the appropriate degree of urgency. There should be established written procedures, which are regularly reviewed and updated, for the organisation of any recall activity. Recall operations should be capable of being initiated promptly down to the required level in the distribution chain. An instruction should be included in the written procedures to store recalled products in a segregated area while their fate is decided. All competent authorities of all countries to which a given product has been distributed should be promptly informed of any intention to recall the product because it is, or is suspected of being, defective. The distribution records should be readily available to the authorized person, and they should contain sufficient information on wholesalers and directly supplied customers to permit an effective recall. The progress of the recall process should be monitored and recorded. Records should include the disposition of the product. A final report should be issued, including a reconciliation between the delivered and recovered quantities of the products. The effectiveness of the arrangements for recalls should be tested and evaluated from time to time.

Self-Inspection and Quality Audits

The purpose of self-inspection is to evaluate the manufacturer's compliance with GMP in all aspects of production and quality control. The self-inspection programme should be designed to detect any shortcomings in the implementation of GMP and to recommend the necessary corrective actions. Self-inspections should be performed routinely, and may be, in addition, performed on special occasions, e.g. in the case of product recalls or repeated rejections, or when an inspection by the health authorities is announced. The team responsible for self-inspection should consist of personnel who can evaluate the implementation of GMP objectively. All recommendations for corrective action should be implemented. The procedure for self-inspection should be documented, and there should be an effective follow-up programme.

Items for Self-Inspection

Written instructions for self-inspection should be established to provide a minimum and uniform standard or requirements. These may include questionnaires on GMP requirements covering at least the following items:

(a) Personnel
(b) Premises including personnel facilities
(c) Maintenance of building and equipment
(d) Storage of starting materials and finished products
(e) Equipment
(f) Production and in-process controls;
(g) Quality control;
(h) Documentation;
(i) Sanitation and hygiene;
(j) Validation and revalidation programme;
(k) Calibration of instruments or measurement systems;
(l) Recall procedures
(m) Complaints management;
(n) Labels control;
(o) Results of previous self-inspection and any corrective steps taken;

Self-Inspection Team

Management should appoint a self-inspection team consisting of experts in their respective fields and familiar with GMP. The members of the team may be appointed from inside or outside the company.

Frequency of Self-Inspection

The frequency at which self-inspection are conducted may depend on company requirements but should preferably be at least once a year. The frequency should be stated in the procedure.

Self-Inspection Report

A report should be made at the completion of a self-inspection. The report should include:

(a) Self-inspection results;

(b) Evaluation and conclusions

(c) Recommended corrective actions.

Follow-up action

There should be an effective follow-up programme. The company management should evaluate both the self-inspection report and the corrective action as necessary.

Quality Audit

It may be useful to supplement self-inspections with a quality audit. A quality audit consists of an examination and assessment of all or part of a quality system with the specific purpose of improving it. A quality audit is usually conducted by outside or independent specialists or a team designated by the management for this purpose. Such audits may also be extended to suppliers and contractors

Supplier's Audits and Approval

The person responsible for quality control should have responsibility together with other relevant departments for approving suppliers who can reliably supply starting and packaging materials that meet established specifications. Before suppliers are approved and included in the approved suppliers list or specifications, they should be evaluated. The evaluation should take into account a supplier's history and the nature of the materials to be supplied. If an audit is required, it should determine the supplier's ability to conform with GMP standards.

CHPATER - 12

Pharmaceutical Packaging and Quality Control Tests of Packaging Materials

Learning Objectives

To learn about

- Pharmaceutical Packaging
- Containers and Closures
- Desirable features of containers and closures
- Types of pharmaceutical packaging
- Packaging Materials
- Glass: Composition and Types
- Manufacture of Glass
- Factors to be considered while selecting Glass as Packaging Materials
- Tests for Glass Containers
- Test for Hydrolytic Resistance (test A)
- Powdered Glass Test (test B)
- Etching Test (test C)
- Water Attack test
- Spectral Transmission test
- Plastic as a Container Material
- Plastic Materials
- (Polythene, Polypropylene, Nylon, Poly Vinyl Chloride, Acrylic multi polymers)
- Properties of Plastics to be considered
- Tests for Plastic
- Leak Test
- Collapsibility Test
- Clarity of Aqueous Extract Test
- Non-Volatile Residue Test

- Biological Test
- Intracutaneous Test
- Eye Irritation Test
- Extraction containers
- Closures
- Rubber Closures
- Tests for Rubber Closures
- Test Procedures
- Light absorption
- Reducing substances
- Volatile sulphides
- Fragmentation test
- Self-seal ability
- Biological Tests
- Extraction containers
- Light absorption

Pharmaceutical Packaging

Pharmaceutical packaging is considered an integral part of the formulation development in the industry and exerts profound impact on the stability of drug product throughout product shelf life. Therefore, pharmaceutical packaging material should have following desirable characteristics. 1) It should protect the drug product from the environmental conditions such as light, reactive gases e.g. oxygen and moisture, 2) It should be compatible with the dosage form and should not interact with any of its components to produce undesirable changes, 3) It should be non-toxic and 4) It should be FDA approved. Selection of packaging material is based upon the type of dosage form, route of administration, chemical nature of the active pharmaceutical ingredients and excipient used in the formulations. Among the factors enlisted, type of dosage form and route of administration significantly affect the selection of container closure system and packaging material as well. For instance, liquid dosage forms are more likely to interact with the packaging materials as compared to solid dosage forms. Moreover, among the liquid dosage forms, non-injectable formulations are less susceptible to interaction with packaging material as compared to the injectable formulations due to significant difference in the preparation techniques.

Containers and Closures

Container

A Pharmaceutical container is a device that holds the drug and may be in direct contact with product. If the container is in direct contact with the drugs it is called an immediate container. (or) It is a device which holds the drug (or) the drug product either directly (or) in an indirect form. In some of the containers product may not be in direct contact with i.e. each unit is packed in a sachet and all of them are stored in containers. Ampoules packed in a container.

Closures

It is a device which protects the drug (or) drug product by preventing the entry of air, moisture, particulate matter, and microorganisms etc., thereby keeping the product in a safe condition and also assists in proper use of the drug.

Desirable Features of Containers and Closures

1. The container must be rigid enough to prevent damage to the contents. e.g. fracture of tablets and crushing of capsules.
2. The materials of construction must not react with contents.
3. The closures must prevent-
   (a) Loss of moisture. e.g. to moisture sensitive tablets and, because their shells are hygroscopic to capsules.
   (b) Loss of moisture from creams and from water-containing ointments and creams.
   (c) Unintentional escape of the content, and
   (d) Entry of direct (or) other contaminants such as odorous vapors that might cause damage to the packaged material.
4. The closure must be easily removed and replaced
5. It must not be difficult to abstract the content (or) empty the container completely.
6. For many products, protection from light must be given.
7. It must be easily to label the container correctly.
8. It must have a pharmaceutical-elegant appearance.
9. They should be inert and should not interact with the drug product.
10. They should have uniform distribution of the product for easy usage and handling.
11. They must be available in form by which they are suitable for a dosage form. eg:- ear drops, nasal drops.
12. They should be able to protect the drug from environment hazards.

13. They should be made in such a way that they have to resist/withstand stocks and abrasions while they are under handling and transport.
14. Containers, used for parental products should be to withstand high sterilization conditions (temperature pressure).
15. The containers used for pharmaceutical purposes should be available in a highly economic rate.
16. Containers used for aerosol packing should be able withstand high pressures.
17. Containers should be available in different size and shapes for easy identification by the patients.

Types of Pharmaceutical Packaging

Packaging is defined as the collection of different components which surrounds the pharmaceutical product from the time of production until its use.

Primary Packaging

This is the first packaging envelope which is in touch with the dosage form or equipment. The packaging needs to be such that there is no interaction with the drug and will provide proper containment of pharmaceuticals. Examples: Blister packages, Strip packages, etc.

Secondary Packaging

This is consecutive covering or package which stores pharmaceuticals packages in it for their grouping. Examples: Cartons, boxes, etc.

Tertiary Packaging

This is to provide bulk handling and shipping of pharmaceuticals from one place to another. Examples: Containers, barrels, etc.

Packaging Materials

Glass

Glass is the most commonly used material in pharmaceutical industries for the packaging of non-injectable liquid formulations. It is used for the fabrication of vials, ampoules, storage bottles, solvent reservoirs etc. Glass contains certain properties, which make it suitable for its use in the packaging of pharmaceutical products. These properties include FDA approval, high strength, ability to modify in different shapes, its crystal-clear appearance, shape and size accessibilities, resistivity towards various chemicals and gases. It can also be flint or coloured based upon their use. Flint glasses or crystal glass is transparent in nature, which enables visual observation of the product. They are rigid, clear, can absorb light of 300 nm wavelength and above and consist of preferably lead and potassium silicates while coloured glass are used to protect the light sensitive pharmaceutical products from photo degradation and hence play a significant role in the stability of such products. Coloured glass usually consists of metal oxides of iron, magnesium etc from which amber or red colour are the choice of containers for pharmaceutical purposes. The major issue with glass containers is the challenge of manufacturing high weight containers and fragile nature of glass.

Composition of Glass

Glass is composed of mainly silica which is added in the form of sand and two or more substances such as soda ash i.e. sodium carbonate, limestone i.e. carbonates of calcium and cullets. Cullets are the broken or melted glass which is added during the manufacturing and act as fusion agents in the containers. Glass also consists of cations such as sodium, potassium, zinc, calcium, barium, and silicon or anion like oxygen. By varying the elemental composition, various properties of the glass can be adjusted according to the use.

The natural glass usually consists of silicon and oxygen tetrahedron wherein each silicon cation is covalently bonded by four oxygen anions and each oxygen anion is bonded with two silicon cations. Introduction of any cation in the glass to improve various properties results in breaking of silicon - oxygen linkage and formation of new electrostatic bonds. These new bonds are weak in nature and hence glass becomes chemically reactive. For instance, addition of more than 12-14% of boric oxide reduces the chemical resistance of glass.

Manufacturing of Glass

Manufacturing of glass is based on its use and type of the container. There are various processes by which glass can be made. Generally, the raw glass materials consisting of sand, soda ash, cullets, limestone etc are melted in hot furnaces at high temperatures i.e. 1500oC for 24 hours. The molten glass is then cooled up to 1000-1200oC. The temperature plays an important role in strength and quality of the container. The cooled glass is then allowed to cast into various shapes by various methods such as blowing, tubing, pressing, drawing etc.

Types of Glasses

Based on surface properties, glass can be classified as Type I, II, III and NP. Type 1 and type II glass are highly resistant and generally considered suitable for the packaging of parenteral pharmaceutical products whereas type III and NP glass are used for the packaging of non-injectable liquids such as oral and topical formulations

Type III

These are simple type of soda lime glass without treatment of the surface with sulphur. It is therefore also known as untreated/regular soda lime glass. Type III glass is generally used for dry powders and the solutions which are not sensitive to alkali i.e. unbuffered solutions or non-aqueous and liquid formulations. Such type of glass is not used for the solutions which are to be sterilized in final containers.

Non-Parenteral Glass

These are general purpose soda lime glass which is used for oral and topical formulations. They are not preferred for the parenteral preparations as most of the alkali release occur from such types of glass.

Factors to be Considered While Selecting Glass as Packaging Materials

While selecting glass as a packaging material for the non-injectable liquid formulations following factors should be considered.

Delamination

Separation of glass sheets from the product contact surface is termed as delamination of glass containers. It results in the appearance of visible flakes in the drug product. Delamination of glass is a major concern in the quality of parenteral drug products.

However, delamination can occur whenever aqueous solution of drugs comes in contact with glass surface. It has also been observed that lack of glass surface integrity produces significant effect on the stability of drugs which is formulated in the form of aqueous solutions. In one study, it was observed that the glass containers negatively influence the stability of drug in solution. They have shown that drug degradation occurred due to the interaction of drug with delaminated glass surfaces within glass container. In another study, it was demonstrated that temperature, terminal sterilization and chemical structure of the drug in solution were the key factors which affect glass durability. They have shown that vials coated with silicon oxide revealed less dissolution of glass as compared to uncoated vials containing glutaric acid, stored at 40°C (4 h at 350°C, two terminal sterilization cycles).

Leaching of Alkali

A glass container mainly constitutes sodium, calcium etc alkali metals. Such alkali metals have a tendency to get leached out from the glass surface.

This process is known as dealkalization and mainly occurs due to attack of water which further leads to removal of alkali from the glass surface or depletion of alkali content from the surface. Dealkalization leads to loss of brilliance and this phenomenon is called as weathering. In case of weathering, the glass surface comes in contact with water. Water has tendency to extract the alkali atoms from the surface which further leads to weakening of bonds leading to loss of brilliance.

This layer can be easily washed by water or weak acid leading to removal or depletion of the alkali atoms. The depleted alkali zone is mainly replaced by the protons and hence an ion exchange phenomenon occurs due to dealkalization process. Dealkalization can also sometimes lead to flaking. The silicon atoms present on the glass surface gets entangled with the water molecules and form silicic acid which further ionizes and hence is responsible for weakening of structure and formation of flakes. It is therefore become important to consider the delamination potential of glass containers for the non-injectable aqueous based liquid formulations.

Photodegradation of Drugs

Some drugs like indomethacin, imipramine, and thyroxine, nifedipine, riboflavin, nitroprussides fluoroquinolones such as ofloxacin (in ointments) undergo degradation on exposure to sunlight. Such types of drugs, if kept in glass containers undergo discoloration, degradation during its shelf life. Glass containers have tendency to absorb visible as well as ultraviolet light. In such cases the container should have property to prevent the light to pass through the surface. Amber coloured glass is preferred over simple glass containers in order to avoid the photo degradation.

Drugs such as doxorubicin undergo photo degradation in clear glass containers but can be prevented using amber coloured glass. Amber colour glass not always prevents the photo degradation. Drugs such as adrenaline can get easily degraded in amber coloured glasses. In such cases plastic containers are more preferred over the coloured glass containers.

Container Size

Container size plays an important role in the stability of pharmaceutical formulation. Container size is inversely proportional to the amount of alkali leached from the containers. This is because of low surface to volume ratio of the container and the solution present in it. If the container is small in size, the area under the contact of alkali increases, thus leaching occurs to a great extent. However, in case of large containers, the surface area with respect to the solution present in the container, so fewer leaching takes place.

Mechanical Properties

Design of the container is also to be taken into consideration. Glass container should be such that it can overcome the heat, hydrolytic degradation. For this purpose, appropriate amount of various metal oxides is to be kept in order to prevent such types of degradation.

Quality of the Container

Container should be such that it retains its quality even after long exposure to sunlight and other environment conditions such as moisture. Cerium oxide is incorporated in glass which prevents the discoloration of the glass, thus maintaining its quality. The surface of glass is treated in order to avoid abrasion and weathering.

Tests for Glass Containers

There are several quality control tests for glass which are performed in order to check its property such as hydrolytic resistance, surface quality etc.

Test for Hydrolytic Resistance: Inner Surface Test (Test A)

This test is performed to evaluate the quality of outer surface of the glass container. The test is performed under controlled conditions with the help of thermocouples, pressure gauge, and autoclave. Quantity of glass containers to be taken for the test is based upon the capacity of the container. Briefly, wash the glass container with distilled water for the prevention of the entry of air bubbles and dry it properly. Fill the containers with carbon dioxide free water and wrap properly with aluminium foils. Place the containers in autoclave within the temperature range of 100-120°C for 20 minutes followed by 120°C for 60 minutes and then 120°C for 40 minutes. Remove the containers out of the autoclave after the equalization of the inside pressure with the atmospheric pressure.

Use methyl red solution as an indicator. Perform the titration using hydrochloric acid [HCl] in burette and compare the end point with the carbon dioxide free water taken as a blank. The volume of HCl required to get the end point is noted and subtracted from the final reading of the blank. The results should not exceed the limits mentioned in the following table (European Pharmacopoeia, 2005)

Table: 12.1 Limits for Hydrolytic test (test A)

Container capacity	No. of containers	Test solution volume (mL)	Volume of 0.020N HCl for Type I or II glass (mL)	Volume of 0.020N HCl for Type III glass (mL)
NMT 1	At least 30	10	2.0	20.0
1-2	At least 20	25	1.8	17.6
2-5	At least 10	50	1.3	13.2
5-10	At least 5	50	1.0	10.2
10-20	At least 5	50	0.80	8.1
20-50	At least 5	60	0.60	6.1
50-100	At least 3	100	0.50	4.8
100-200	At least 3	100	0.40	3.8
200-500	At least 3	100	0.30	2.9
>500	At least 3	100	0.20	2.2

*(European Pharmacopoeia, 2005).

Powdered Glass Test: Glass Grain Test (Test B):

Take three out of all the containers, rinse and dry them. Crush the containers into coarse fragments and transfer them to the mortar. Pass the crushed fragments through sieves 710(μm) and 425(μm) and sift properly. Separate the fragments retained by sieve 710(μm). Glass fragments obtained on sieve 425(μm) are taken for further procedure. Magnets can be used for removal of metals such as iron. These glass fragments can also be suspended in acetone to remove metal impurities. Immerse the glass fragments completely in acetone, wash and dry.

Take the fragments out of the dried glass fragments, in conical flask with carbon dioxide free water and titrate with HCl. Compare with the blank containing only carbon dioxide free water. Perform the hydrolytic tests. The limit is same as test A with same limits (European Pharmacopoeia 5.0, 2005).

Etching Test: Surface Treatment Test (Test C)

This test is performed to check whether the surface of container is treated or not i.e. to differentiate between Type II and III. Select and rinse the containers with distilled water, hydrofluoric acid and hydrochloric acid in ratio 1:9. Wash the containers several times with water and perform test A. If the values exceed the limits of test A, then it is concluded that glass containers are surface treated (European Pharmacopoeia 5.0, 2005).

Water Attack Test

This test is performed for the treated glass containers, i.e., type-II glass. The treated glass container loses its resistivity to chemicals, solvents if they are repeatedly subjected to autoclaving. Water attack test is generally performed in order to check the alkali limits in the treated glass containers. Rinse and dry the glass containers with purified water. Fill the container with the purified water free from carbon dioxide and seal them properly with aluminium foils. Subject these containers to autoclave for temperature 121 degrees Celsius for 60 minutes. Take the containers out of the autoclave on the equalization of the pressure. Take 100 mL of this content in 250 mL conical flask and add methyl red solution as an indicator. Titrate the solution with 0.02 N sulphuric acid and observe the end point. Compare the end point of the test solution with that of blank and subtract the blank reading from it. The volume limits of 0.02 N sulphuric acid for type-2 glass with capacity of 100 mL or less should not exceed 0.7 and 0.2 for more than 100 mL (United States Pharmacopoeia USP 38 and National Formulary NF 33).

Spectral Transmission

Spectral transmission is done using UV- VIS spectrophotometer. Cut the Glass with uniform wall thickness and place into a holder. Carefully rinse and dry the pieces. Cover the holder properly with an opaque paper. The glass pieces (specimen) should have more length than the slit. Mount the specimen carefully and kept in the UV-VIS Spectrophotometer. Pass the beam of light in such a manner that it is perpendicular to the surface of specimen. Measure the transmission in region of 290-450 nm. The containers for the parenteral purposes should not exceed the limits mentioned in the table below (European Pharmacopoeia 5.0, 2005, United States Pharmacopoeia USP 38 and National Formulary NF 33).

Table 12.2 Limits for the Spectral transmission test*

Maximum percentage of spectral transmission at any wavelength between 250-450 nm		
	Flame-sealed containers	**Containers with closures**
1	50	25
2	45	20
3-5	40	15
6-10	35	13
11-20	30	12
More than 20	25	10

*(European Pharmacopoeia, 2005). General Tests and Assays. In United States Pharmacopoeia and National Formulary.

Plastic as a Container Material

Plastic is also widely used for the construction of whole body of the container or a part of the containers. Bottles, bags and tubes are the most commonly used plastic based containers. Moreover, inner side of the metal tubes sometime is also coated with plastic to prevent the interaction between the content of the container and the metal. Plastic based closures are also used for the packaging of pharmaceutical products.

Plastic as a packaging material offer several advantages including unbreakable nature light weight, ability to form different shaped containers, flexibility and durability. Plastic is made from cross linking of synthetic or semi synthetic long chain polymers. High durability and flexibility of the material are due to the cross-linked polymeric structures. Certain additives are also added with the building block polymers to improve the various physicochemical properties of the material. In general, different additives include antioxidants, antistatic agents, colours, impact modifiers, lubricants, plasticizers and stabilize.

Plastic has a tendency to develop a static charge on the surface because of its insulating nature which further is responsible for the attraction of dust particles on the surface of plastic making it dull in appearance and contaminate. Additives such as long chain aliphatic amines, phosphate esters act as antistatic agents which prevents this charge to develop on plastic surface. Fillers are used to add to the strength of the plastic and to increase the bulk quantity of the whole plastic material. Plastics have a tendency to permeate oxygen through its surface hence oxygen reacts with the plastic surface, breaks its polymerized long chain structure and react with them which leads to oxidation of the material, hence additives such as antioxidants like phenolic compounds are used to prevent oxidation. Antimicrobials such as silver ion based Microblok are added for prevention from the microbial attack. Increasing the shear stress, plastic may get deformed and cracked.

To prevent this damage, impact modifiers such as acrylic impact modifiers, paraloid are added to increase its strength. Reinforcing agents such as glass fibres and metal powders are added to plastics in order to improve the tensile strength of plastic material.

Plastics melt while processing for smooth flow ability and to mould plastic in various forms. Thus, processing aids like fluoropolymers is used to increase the flow ability of plastic for easy conversion of plastics in variety of forms. Plastics made from simple long chain polymerization are less flexible, thus it is the role of plasticizers such as di-Ethylhexyl phthalate to increase its flexibility. Light stabilizers such as HALS (hindered amine light stabilizers) are available which prevents the photo degradation of the product. Lubricants are added to improve the process of manufacturing of plastic by increasing the flow ability.

Integrity of the plastic depends on the chemical structure of the copolymers bonded together, molecular weight of the plastic, orientation of the molecules, linkage pattern of the copolymers as well as additives present in the plastic.

Plastic Materials

Polyethylene

Polyethylene is the most widely used material in fabrication of plastic containers for pharmaceutical purpose. Excellent barrier for moisture and resistance to the attack of strong acids and alkali are the two major advantages of polyethylene while lack of transparency and highly permeable to oxygen, odours and flavours are major limitation of this class of material with respect to their use in pharmaceutical packaging. Based upon density, polyethylene can be classified in two type's namely high density and low-density polyethylene. As the density increases, material become less permeable to reactive gases and hence high-density polyethylene is generally preferred over low density material for the packaging of oxygen sensitive. Antioxidants are generally added to these polymers to prevent oxidation during processing. Generally used antioxidants are butylated hydroxy toluene or dilauryl thio-dipropionate. Antistatic agents such as polyethylene glycol and long chain fatty amides are added to bottle grade polyethylene to minimize the accumulation of dust at the surface of bottles during packaging and storage.

Polypropylene

Polypropylene is resistant to various chemicals/solvents and heat hence suitable for the packaging of the products which need to be sterilized. However, it is sensitive to hot aromatic solvents and become soften when come in contact with these chemicals. Unlike low density polyethylene, polypropylene is less permeable to reactive gases like oxygen or vapor. The only disadvantage of the material is that polypropylene become brittle at low temperature and need to be mixed with polyethylene to overcome this problem.

Nylon

Nylon is a polyamide-based material and generally used in the fabrication of thin walled containers. Nylon based containers can be sterilized by autoclave. Nylon is also resistant to strong acids and alkali as well as various organic and inorganic chemicals. It provides strong barrier to oxygen while it is highly permeable to moisture. It also has a high potential of interaction with the drugs and hence not preferred when the long-term storage of drug products is required.

Polyvinylchloride

Polyvinylchloride is used to construct plastic bottles and lamination of inner side of the glass bottles for the packaging of liquid formulations. PVC offers several advantages including rigid, transparent, and stiff in nature. Incorporation of plasticizer in the PVC reduces the rigidity. It is also sensitive to heat and ultraviolent light. To improve the stability of PVC towards temperature and radiations, stabilizers need to be incorporated. Generally used stabilizers to improve the stability of PVC are dioctyl-tin-marcapto acetate, sulphur, calcium and zinc salts and calcium-zinc stabilization materials. PVC is impermeable to fixed and volatile alcohols, oxygen and moisture. PVC is resistant to acids and alkali but sensitive to oxidizing agents.

Acrylic Multipolymers

It has several advantages like rigid, transparent, resistant to wide range of chemicals, impermeable to oxygen and cost effective. It is found to be suitable for the packaging of wide range of products including sterile and non-sterile liquid formulations.

Other Plastic Materials

Other materials like polystyrene, polyterpthalate [PET] and polycarbonates are also used in the packaging of pharmaceutical products however; these materials are not used for the packaging of non-injectable liquid formulations. For instance, polystyrene is used for the packaging of solid oral dosage form and dry formulations, PET is used to prepare of packaging films and plastic bottles for the carbonated beverages and polycarbonate is used for the packaging of sterile products.

Properties of Plastics to be Considered

Sorption

Sorption is characterized as the loss of formulation constituents due to the interaction with packaging materials. A sorption phenomenon is more prominent in liquid formulations as compared to the solid dosage forms. Sorption of drugs from the liquid formulations leads to significance decrease in drug content of the formulations and subsequently affects the therapeutic efficacy of the drug. Martens HJ et al. demonstrated that Diazepam, isosorbide dinitrate, nitroglycerin, and warfarin sodium showed significant sorption of drugs when stored in the dark at room temperature for 24 h in PVC bags while there was no loss of drug content observed when the same formulations were stored in glass bottles and clear flex. In another study, decrease in concentration of diazepam and nitroglycerin was observed within 4 h at room temperature in PVC containers whereas no change in concentration of drugs was observed in glass bottles and polyethylene containers Sorption influxes not only the drug content of the formulation but also responsible for the loss of preservatives and pigments from the liquid formulation which subsequently affects the stability as well as performance of the formulation. Significant loss of propyl and butylparaben in oral solutions packaged in PET bottles has been observed. Preservative concentration and temperature influenced the sorption of parabens by the PET. Sorption of pigments by low density polyethylene containers has been reported Factors which affect the sorption by packaging material are pH of the formulation, chemical structure and concentration of the drug, type of packaging material, temperature and contact duration.

Photo Degradation

Many active pharmaceutical ingredients degrade when exposed to the ultra-violet [UV] light. This phenomenon is termed as photodegradation of the drugs. Presence of specific functional groups in most polymers like carbonyl and aromatic rings are prone to absorb UV radiations and increase the transmittance of the plastic container towards UV radiations. Moreover, absorption of UV radiation also results in the change in physical and chemical properties of the plastic containers which subsequently affect the stability of the drugs in formulations. Opacifying agents are generally added to the plastic containers to prevent the photodegradation of the light sensitive drugs. Lamination of plastic containers by aluminium foils and use of light resistant secondary packaging materials are the other options to prevent the photo degradation.

Desorption

One or more additives are added in the plastic materials to impart specific properties to the plastic. This additive provides possibility of leaching or migration from the containers to the formulations. Migration of the colouring agents from the plastic containers to the liquid formulations is an example of leaching or desorption of additives. Factors which generally affect the desorption are pH, temperature, solvent type and type of plastic material and additive present in the plastic materials.

Permeation

Plastic materials may provide passage to the gases and water vapor and leads to the instability of the packaged formulations. Permeation of oxygen and water vapours through packaging material can be a serious concern for the stability of oxidation and hydrolysis sensitive drugs respectively. Storage conditions like temperature and humidity significantly affect the permeation of gases and vapor and permeation increases with increase in temperature. Type of materials also affects the permeation for instance, nylon provides poor barrier to water vapours as compared to polyethylene. Method of manufacturing and type of additives also affects the permeation of plastic based packaging containers. Permeation of volatile oils from the formulations packaged in the plastic containers affect the aroma of the formulation.

Physical stability of the formulation is also affected by the permeation. Certain oil in water type emulsions have shown the permeation of oils from the formulation to the package in hydrophobic plastic containers.

Tests for Plastic

Leak Test

The test is performed to check for any leakage from the container. Invert 10 filled closed containers of water at room temperature for 24 hours. No leakage observed from the container indicates the container is fit for use (Welfare, 2007, United States Pharmacopoeia USP 38 and National Formulary NF 33).

Collapsibility Test

Collapsibility test is performed in order to check the squeezing property of the container. Take container with the required contents. Squeeze the contents with optimum force. 90% of the content extruded indicates at optimum force and temperature indicated the container is fit for use (Welfare, 2007, United States Pharmacopoeia USP 38 and National Formulary NF 33).

Clarity of Aqueous Extract Test

Cut several strips of 20cmsq area from both the sides from the container to be tested. The strips should be taken from the area of the container that is unlabelled, unmarked, and non- laminated. Wash the strips twice with distilled water. Select about 60-65 strips from the washed strips and transfer them in cleaned conical flask of 250mL. Add water to the conical flask and keep for autoclave for 120oC for 30 minutes. Carry out the same procedure for the blank containing water. Cool the strips and compare the test with the blank for the clarity (Welfare, 2007, United States Pharmacopoeia USP 38 and National Formulary NF 33).

Non-Volatile Residue Test

Take 100mL of extract from the clarity extract solution and heat it to dryness till the constant weight is obtained. The residue obtained should not be more than 12.5 mg (Welfare, 2007, United States Pharmacopoeia USP 38 and National Formulary NF 33).

Biological Test

Biological test is performed to check the compatibility of the container with the humans. The plastic should not react with the solution to cause toxic problems. Prepare the extract and the blank and dilute with PEG 400 and 4.1 volumes of sodium chloride injections respectively. Keep the solutions in the type 2 glass container. Agitate the solution properly before withdrawing it with the help of injection.

Table 12.3 General Considerations of Biological test*

Blank	Animal	Route	Dose/Kg As per IP	Dose/Kg As per USP
NaCl Injection	Mice	IV	50 mL	50 mL
NaCl + 5% v/v ethanol	Mice	IV	50mL	50mL
PEG 400	Mice	IP	10g	10g
Vegetable oil	Mice	IP	50mL	50mL

*(Welfare, 2007; General Tests and Assays. In United States Pharmacopoeia and National Formulary).

Take healthy albino mice weighing 17-23g and group them in test and blank. Inject the extracted sample in the test group and blank in the blank group. Observe the mice for 0, 4, and so on till 72 hours. Compare the test group with the blank for any reactivity. If two or more mice die, continue the test with 10 more mice. The fitness of plastic is indicated if no single mice undergo reactivity. General considerations for the biological tests including route of administration dose and blank is summarized in table 12.3 (Welfare, 2007, United States Pharmacopoeia USP 38 and National Formulary NF 33).

Intracutaneous Test

It is done in order to find any local toxicity if occurred due to the reactivity of the container with the product. Take three rabbits for each sample to be tested. Remove the hairs from the surface to be examined and clean it with dilute ethanol. Inject or use an implant to be tested of test and blank on same animal at two different sites. Observe and compare the local area for the edema, erythema and necrosis of test with that of blank. Compare the limits by calculating the score for the local toxicities according to the tables given below. (Welfare, 2007, United States Pharmacopoeia USP 38 and National Formulary NF 33).

Table 12.4 Score for erythema and eschar formation*

Erythema and eschar Formation	Score	
	As per IP	As per USP
No erythema	0	0
Very slight erythema	1	1
Well-defined erythema	2	2
Moderate to severe erythema	3	3
Severe erythema to slight	4	4

(Welfare, 2007; General Tests and Assays. In United States Pharmacopoeia and National Formulary)

Table 12.5 Score for edema formation*

Edema formation	Score	
	As per IP	As per USP
No edema	0	0
Very slight edema	1	1
Slight edema	2	2
Moderate edema	3	3
Severe edema	4	4

*(Welfare, 2007; General Tests and Assays. In United States Pharmacopoeia and National Formulary)

Eye Irritation Test

Select healthy rabbits for the test and examine it properly. Restrain the animal and instill 100µL of sterile water for injection as blank in one eye and the sample extract to be tested in another eye. Observe the animal for 24, 48 and 72 hours. Compare the test for irritation with respect to blank.

Closures

Rubber Closures

A closure for a container for an aqueous parenteral preparation or for a sterile powder is a packaging component which is in direct contact with the drug. A rubber closure is made of materials obtained by vulcanisation (cross-linking) of elastomers with appropriate additives. The elastomers are produced from natural or synthetic substances by polymerisation, polyaddition or polycondensation. The nature of the principal components and of the various additives such as vulcanisers, accelerators, stabilising agents, pigments, etc. depends on the properties required for the finished closure.

Rubber closures are used in a number of formulations and consequently different closures possess different properties. The closures chosen for use with a particular preparation should be such that the components of the preparation in contact with the closure are not adsorbed onto the surface of the closure to an extent sufficient to affect the product adversely. The closure should not yield to the product substances in quantities sufficient to affect its stability or to present a risk of toxicity. The closures should be compatible with the preparation for which they are used throughout the shelf-life of the product. It is impracticable to devise a set of standards which, if complied with, will ensure the compatibility of any closure with the preparation for which it is to be used. A compatibility test has, therefore, to be carried out before a rubber mix is approved. The user of the closures must obtain an assurance from the supplier that the composition of the closure does not vary from supply to supply and that it is identical to that of the closure used during compatibility testing. When the user is informed of changes in the composition, compatibility testing must be repeated, totally or partly depending on the nature of the changes.

Tests for Rubber Closures

Test Procedures

The following test procedures apply to rubber closures which comprise wads (flat rubber discs), plugs (with or without skirt or flange) and caps (rubber covers held in position on the outsides of the containers by the tension of the rubber) so as to form with their appropriate seals an effective barrier against micro-organisms after sterilisation. Identification of the type of rubber used for closures is not covered in the following tests. The tests given distinguish elastomer and non-elastomer closures but do not differentiate the various types of rubber.

Description. Rubber closures are elastic and either translucent or opaque; the colour depends on the additives used. They are homogeneous and practically free from flash and adventitious materials such as fibres, foreign particles and adhering rubber pieces.

Identification A. Heat 1 g to 2 g in a heat-resistant test-tube over an open flame to dry the sample and continue heating until the vapours formed are condensed near the top edge of the test-tube. Deposit a few drops of the condensate on a potassium bromide disc and examine by infrared absorption spectrophotometry (2.4.6), comparing with the spectrum obtained with the type (standard) sample. B. The total ash (2.3.19) is within ± 10 per cent of the value obtained with the type sample.

Preparation of Samples

Wash the closures by agitation in a 0.2 per cent w/v solution of an anionic surface-active agent for 5 minutes at room temperature. Rinse five times with water, place a number of the washed closures corresponding to a surface area of about 100 cm2, in a suitable container of borosilicate glass or inert material, add 200 mL of water per 100 cm2, surface area of the closures and weigh. Cover the mouth of the container with aluminium foil or a borosilicate glass beaker and heat in an autoclave so that a temperature of 119° to 123° is reached within 20 to 30 minutes and maintain at that temperature for 30 minutes. Cool to room temperature over about 30 minutes and make up to the original weight with water for injection. Shake and immediately separate the solution from the closures by decantation (Solution A)

Appearance of Solution

Solution A is not more opalescent than opalescence standard OS3 (2.4.1, IP), and not more intensely coloured than reference solution BYS6 (2.4.1, IP).

pH of Aqueous Extract

To 20 mL of solution A add 0.1 mL of bromothymol blue solution. Not more than 0.3 mL of 0.01M sodium hydroxide or 0.8 mL of 0.01M hydrochloric acid is required to change the colour of the solution to blue or yellow respectively.

Light Absorption

Carry out the test within 4 hours of preparing solution A. Filter solution A through a membrane filter with a nominal pore size of 0.5 μm and reject the first few mL of the filtrate. Measure the light absorption of the filtrate in the range 220 to 360 nm (2.4.7), using as the blank a solution prepared in the same manner as solution A but using 200 mL of water without the closures. The absorbance is not more than 2.0; if necessary, dilute the filtrate before measurement and correct the results for the dilution.

Reducing Substances

Carry out the test within 4 hours of preparing solution A. To 20 mL of solution A, add 1 mL of 1M sulphuric acid and 20 mL of 0.002 M potassium permanganate and boil for 3 minutes. Cool, add 1g of potassium iodide and titrate immediately with 0.01 M sodium thiosulphate using 0.25 mL of starch solution, added towards the end of the titration, as indicator. Repeat the operation using 20 mL of the blank prepared in the test for Light absorption. The difference between the titration volumes is not more than 7.0 mL.

Heavy Metals (2.3.13)

20 mL of solution A complies with the limit test for heavy metals, Method A.

Residue on Evaporation

Evaporate 50 mL of solution A to dryness on a water-bath and dry at 105°. The residue weighs not more than 4.0 mg.

Volatile Sulphides

Place closures, cut if necessary, with a total surface area of 20 ± 2 cm2 in a 100-mL conical flask and add 50 mL of a 2 per cent w/v solution of citric acid. Place a piece of lead acetate paper over the mouth of the flask and maintain the paper in position by placing over it an inverted weighing bottle. Heat in an autoclave at 121 ± 2° for 30 minutes. Any black stain on the paper is not more intense than that of a standard prepared at the same time in the same manner using 0.154 mg of sodium sulphide and 50 mL of a 2 per cent w/v solution of citric acid. **Sterilisation test.** The closures 'prepared' in the aforementioned manner shall not soften or become tacky and there shall be no visual change in the closure.

Fragmentation Test

This test is applicable to closures intended to be pierced by a hypodermic needle. For closures that are intended to be used for aqueous preparations, place a volume of water corresponding to the nominal volume minus 4 mL in each of 12 clean vials, close the vials with the 'prepared' closures, secure with a cap and allow to stand for 16 hours. For closures that are intended to be used for dry preparations, close 12 clean vials with the 'prepared' closures. Using a lubricated, long-bevel (bevel angle of 10° to 14°) hypodermic needle with an external diameter of 0.8 mm (21 SWG) fitted to a clean syringe, inject 1 mL of water into the vial and remove 1 mL of air; carry out this operation 4 times for each closure, piercing each time at a different site. Use a new needle for each closure and check that the needle is not blunted during the test. Pass the liquid in the vials through a filter with a nominal pore size of 0.5 µm. Count the number of fragments visible to the naked eye. The total number of fragments is not more than 10 except in the case of butyl rubber closures where the total number of fragments is not more than 15.

Self-Sealability

This test is applicable to closures intended to be used with multidose containers. Fill 10 suitable vials with water to the nominal volume, close the vials with the 'prepared' closures and secure with a cap. For each closure, use a new hypodermic needle with an external diameter of 0.8 mm (21 SWG) and pierce the closure 10 times, piercing each time at a different site. Immerse the vials upright in a 0.1 per cent w/v solution of methylene blue and reduce the external pressure by 27kPa for 10 minutes. Restore the atmospheric pressure and leave the vials immersed for 30 minutes. Rinse the outside of the vials. None of the vials contains any trace of coloured solution.

Biological Tests

The following tests may be done when the compatibility test is done for approving a rubber mix for the manufacture of closures and whenever the composition of the rubber mix is altered. The tests are designed to evaluate the biological response in test animals of an extract of the closures. The contact of the extracting medium with the total surface of the closures, the time and temperature during extraction and the aseptic handling and storage of the extract are important. Particular care must be exercised in the preparation of the extract to be injected to prevent contamination with microorganisms and foreign matter.

Extraction Containers

Use only containers such as screw capped culture test-tubes or bottles, of Type I glass. Screw caps should have suitable elastomeric liners and the exposed surface of the liner should be completely protected with an inert solid disc, 50 to 75 μm in thickness, and fabricated from a material such as teflon or any other polytetrafluoroethylene resin. All glassware should be thoroughly rinsed with chromic acid mixture, followed by prolonged rinsing with sterile water for injection. Containers and devices used for extraction, transfer of administration of test material should be sterile and dried by a suitable process.

Appearance of Solution

Solution A is not more opalescent than opalescence standard OS3 (2.4.1), and not more intensely coloured than reference solution BYS6 (2.4.1). pH of aqueous extract. To 20 mL of solution A add 0.1 mL of bromothymol blue solution. Not more than 0.3 mL of 0.01M sodium hydroxide or 0.8 mL of 0.01M hydrochloric acid is required to change the colour of the solution to blue or yellow respectively.

Light Absorption

Carry out the test within 4 hours of preparing solution A. Filter solution A through a membrane filter with a nominal pore size of 0.5 μm and reject the first few mL of the filtrate. Measure the light absorption of the filtrate in the range 220 to 360 nm (2.4.7), using as the blank a solution prepared in the same manner as solution A but using 200 mL of water without the closures. The absorbance is not more than 2.0; if necessary, dilute the filtrate before measurement and correct the results for the dilution. Reducing substances. Carry out the test within 4 hours of preparing solution A. To 20 mL of solution A, add 1 mL of 1M sulphuric acid and 20 mL of 0.002 M potassium permanganate and boil for 3 minutes. Cool, add 1g of potassium iodide and titrate immediately with 0.01 M sodium thiosulphate using 0.25 mL of starch solution, added towards the end of the titration, as indicator. Repeat the operation using 20 mL of the blank prepared in the test for Light absorption. The difference between the titration volumes is not more than 7.0 mL. Heavy Metals (2.3.13). 20 mL of solution A complies with the limit test for heavy metals, Method A. Residue on evaporation: Evaporate 50 mL of solution A to dryness on a water-bath and dry at 105°. The residue weighs not more than 4.0 mg. Volatile sulphides. Place closures, cut if necessary, with a total surface area of 20 ± 2 cm2 in a 100-mL conical flask and add 50 mL of a 2 per cent w/v solution of citric acid. Place a piece of lead acetate paper over the mouth of the flask and maintain the paper in position by placing over it an inverted weighing bottle. Heat in an autoclave at 121 ± 2° for 30 minutes. Any black stain on the paper is not more intense than that of a standard prepared at the same time in the same manner using 0.154 mg of sodium sulphide and 50 mL of a 2 per cent w/v solution of citric acid. Sterilisation test. The closures 'prepared' in the afore mentioned manner shall not soften or become tacky and there shall be no visual change in the closure. Fragmentation test. This test is applicable to closures intended to be pierced by a hypodermic needle. For closures that are intended to be used for aqueous preparations, place a volume of water corresponding to the nominal volume minus 4 mL in each of 12 clean vials, close the vials with the 'prepared' closures, secure with a cap and allow to stand for 16 hours. For closures that are intended to be used for dry preparations, close 12 clean vials with the 'prepared' closures. Using a lubricated, long-bevel (bevel angle of 10° to 14°) hypodermic needle with an external diameter of 0.8 mm (21 SWG) fitted to a clean syringe, inject 1 mL of water into the vial and remove 1 mL of air; carry out this operation 4 times for each closure, piercing each time at a different site. Use a new needle for each closure and check that the needle is not blunted during the test. Pass the liquid in the vials through a filter with a nominal pore size of 0.5 μm. Count the number of fragments visible to the naked eye. The total number of fragments is not more than 10 except in the case of butyl rubber closures where the total number of fragments is not more than 15. Self-sealability. This test is applicable to closures intended to be used with multidose containers. Fill 10 suitable vials with water to the nominal volume, close the vials with the 'prepared' closures and secure with a cap. For each closure, use a new hypodermic needle with an external diameter of 0.8 mm (21 SWG) and pierce the closure 10 times, piercing each time at a different site. Immerse the vials upright in a 0.1 per cent w/v solution of methylene blue and reduce the external pressure by 27kPa for 10 minutes. Restore the atmospheric pressure and leave the vials immersed for 30 minutes. Rinse the outside of the vials. None of the vials contains any trace of coloured solution. Biological Tests The following tests may be done when the compatibility test is done for approving a rubber mix for the manufacture of closures and whenever the composition of the rubber mix is altered. The tests are designed to evaluate the biological response in test animals of an extract of the closures. The contact of the extracting medium with the total surface of the closures, the time and temperature during extraction and the aseptic handling and storage of the extract are important. Particular care must be exercised in the preparation of the extract to be injected to prevent contamination with microorganisms and foreign matter. Extraction containers. Use only containers such as screw capped culture test-tubes or bottles, of Type I glass. Screw caps should have suitable elastomeric liners and the exposed surface of the liner should be completely protected with an inert solid disc, 50 to 75 μm in thickness, and fabricated from a material such as Teflon or any other polytetrafluoroethylene resin. All glassware should be thoroughly rinsed with chromic acid mixture, followed by prolonged rinsing with sterile water for injection. Containers and devices used for extraction, transfer of administration of test material should be sterile and dried by a suitable process.

CHPATER - 13

Good Laboratory Practices (GLP)

Learning Objectives

To learn about

- General Provisions of GLP
- Definitions
- Inspection of a Testing Facility:
- Organization and Personnel:
- Personnel
- Testing Facility Management
- Study Director
- Quality Assurance Unit
- Facilities
- Animal Care Facilities
- Animal Supply Facilities
- Facilities for Handling Test and Control Articles
- Laboratory Operation Areas
- Specimen and Data Storage Facilities
- Equipment
- Maintenance and Calibration of Equipment
- Testing Facilities Operation
- Reagents and Solutions
- Animal Care
- Test and Control Articles
- Test and Control Article Handling
- Protocol for and Conduct of a Non-Clinical Laboratory Study
- Records and Reports
- Disqualification of Testing Facilities
- Grounds for Disqualification

- Final Order on Disqualification
- Action Upon Disqualification
- Alternative or Additional Actions to Disqualification
- Suspension or Termination of a Testing Facility by a Sponsor
- Reinstatement of a Disqualified Testing Facility

Introduction (General Provisions)

Good laboratory practices (GLP) describe guidelines for conducting nonclinical laboratory studies that support or are intended to support applications for research or marketing permits for products regulated by the Food and Drug Administration, including food and color additives, animal food additives, human and animal drugs, medical devices for human use, biological products, and electronic products.

Definitions

As used in this part, the following terms shall have the meanings specified:

1. **Test article** means any food additive, color additive, drug, biological product, electronic product, medical device for human use.
2. **Control article** means any food additive, color additive, drug, biological product, electronic product, medical device for human use, or any article other than a test article, feed, or water that is administered to the test system in the course of a nonclinical laboratory study for the purpose of establishing a basis for comparison with the test article.
3. **Nonclinical laboratory study** means *in vivo* or *in vitro* experiments in which test articles are studied prospectively in test systems under laboratory conditions to determine their safety. The term does not include studies utilizing human subjects or clinical studies or field trials in animals. The term does not include basic exploratory studies carried out to determine whether a test article has any potential utility or to determine physical or chemical characteristics of a test article.
4. **Sponsor means:**
    1. A person who initiates and supports, by provision of financial or other resources, a nonclinical laboratory study;
    2. A person who submits a nonclinical study to the Food and Drug Administration in support of an application for a research or marketing permit; or
    3. A testing facility, if it both initiates and actually conducts the study.

5. **Testing facility** means a person who actually conducts a nonclinical laboratory study, i.e., actually uses the test article in a test system. Testing facility includes any establishment that conducts nonclinical laboratory studies and any consulting laboratory that conducts such studies. Testing facility encompasses only those operational units that are being or have been used to conduct nonclinical laboratory studies.
   Person includes an individual, partnership, corporation, association, scientific or academic establishment, government agency, or organizational unit thereof, and any other legal entity.
6. **Test system** means any animal, plant, microorganism, or subparts thereof to which the test or control article is administered or added for study. Test system also includes appropriate groups or components of the system not treated with the test or control articles.
7. **Raw data** means any laboratory worksheets, records, memoranda, notes, or exact copies thereof, that are the result of original observations and activities of a nonclinical laboratory study and are necessary for the reconstruction and evaluation of the report of that study. Raw data may include photographs, microfilm or microfiche copies, computer printouts, magnetic media, including dictated observations, and recorded data from automated instruments.
8. **Quality assurance unit** means any person or organizational element, except the study director, designated by testing facility management to perform the duties relating to quality assurance of nonclinical laboratory studies.
9. **Study director means** the individual responsible for the overall conduct of a nonclinical laboratory study.

Inspection of a Testing Facility

(a) A testing facility shall permit an authorized employee of the Food and Drug Administration, at reasonable times and in a reasonable manner, to inspect the facility and to inspect (and in the case of records also to copy) all records and specimens required to be maintained regarding studies within the scope of this part. The records inspection and copying requirements shall not apply to quality assurance unit records of findings and problems, or to actions recommended and taken.

(b) The Food and Drug Administration will not consider a nonclinical laboratory study in support of an application for a research or marketing permit if the testing facility refuses to permit inspection. The determination that a nonclinical laboratory study will not be considered in support of an application for a research or marketing permit does not, however, relieve the applicant for such a permit of any obligation under any applicable statute or regulation to submit the results of the study to the Food and Drug Administration.

Organization and Personnel

Personnel

(i) Each individual engaged in the conduct of study are responsible for the supervision of a nonclinical laboratory study shall have education, training, and experience, or combination thereof, to enable that individual to perform the assigned functions.

(ii) Each testing facility shall maintain a current summary of training and experience and job description for each individual engaged in or supervising the conduct of a nonclinical laboratory study.

(iii) There shall be a sufficient number of personnel for the timely and proper conduct of the study according to the protocol.

(iv) Personnel shall take necessary personal sanitation and health precautions designed to avoid contamination of test and control articles and test systems.

(v) Personnel engaged in a nonclinical laboratory study shall wear clothing appropriate for the duties they perform. Such clothing shall be changed as often as necessary to prevent microbiological, radiological, or chemical contamination of test systems and test and control articles.

(vi) Any individual found at any time to have an illness that may adversely affect the quality and integrity of the nonclinical laboratory study shall be excluded from direct contact with test systems, test and control articles and any other operation or function that may adversely affect the study until the condition is corrected. All personnel shall be instructed to report to their immediate supervisors any health or medical conditions that may reasonably be considered to have an adverse effect on a nonclinical laboratory study.

Testing Facility Management

For each nonclinical laboratory study, testing facility management shall:

(a) Designate a study director before the study is initiated.

(b) Replace the study director promptly if it becomes necessary to do so during the conduct of a study.

(c) Assure that there is a quality assurance unit

(d) Assure that test and control articles or mixtures have been appropriately tested for identity, strength, purity, stability, and uniformity, as applicable.

(e) Assure that personnel, resources, facilities, equipment, materials, and methodologies are available as scheduled.

(f) Assure that personnel clearly understand the functions they are to perform.

(g) Assure that any deviations from these regulations reported by the quality assurance unit are communicated to the study director and corrective actions are taken and documented.

Study Director

For each nonclinical laboratory study, a scientist or other professional of appropriate education, training, and experience, or combination thereof, shall be identified as the study director. The study director has overall responsibility for the technical conduct of the study, as well as for the interpretation, analysis, documentation and reporting of results, and represents the single point of study control. The study director shall assure that:

(a) The protocol, including any change, is approved and is followed.

(b) All experimental data, including observations of unanticipated responses of the test system are accurately recorded and verified.

(c) Unforeseen circumstances that may affect the quality and integrity of the nonclinical laboratory study are noted when they occur, and corrective action is taken and documented.

(d) Test systems are as specified in the protocol.

(e) All applicable good laboratory practice regulations are followed.

(f) All raw data, documentation, protocols, specimens, and final reports are transferred to the archives during or at the close of the study.

Quality Assurance Unit

(a) A testing facility shall have a quality assurance unit which shall be responsible for monitoring each study to assure management that the facilities, equipment, personnel, methods, practices, records, and controls are in conformance with the regulations. For any given study, the quality assurance unit shall be entirely separate from and independent of the personnel engaged in the direction and conduct of that study.

(b) The quality assurance unit shall

1. Maintain a copy of a master schedule sheet of all nonclinical laboratory studies conducted at the testing facility indexed by test article and containing the test system, nature of study, date study was initiated, current status of each study, identity of the sponsor, and name of the study director.
2. Maintain copies of all protocols pertaining to all nonclinical laboratory studies for which the unit is responsible.
3. Inspect each nonclinical laboratory study at intervals adequate to assure the integrity of the study and maintain written and properly signed records of each periodic inspection showing the date of the inspection, the study inspected, the phase or segment of the study inspected, the person performing the inspection, findings and problems, action recommended and taken to resolve existing problems, and any scheduled date for reinspection. Any problems found during the course of an inspection which are likely to affect study integrity shall be brought to the attention of the study director and management immediately.
4. Periodically submit to management and the study director written status reports on each study, noting any problems and the corrective actions taken.
5. Determine that no deviations from approved protocols or standard operating procedures were made without proper authorization and documentation.
6. Review the final study report to assure that such report accurately describes the methods and standard operating procedures, and that the reported results accurately reflect the raw data of the nonclinical laboratory study.
7. Prepare and sign a statement to be included with the final study report which shall specify the dates inspections were made and findings reported to management and to the study director.

(c) The responsibilities and procedures applicable to the quality assurance unit, the records maintained by the quality assurance unit, and the method of indexing such records shall be in writing and shall be maintained.

(d) A designated representative of the Food and Drug Administration shall have access to the written procedures established for the inspection.

Facilities

Each testing facility shall be of suitable size and construction to facilitate the proper conduct of nonclinical laboratory studies. It shall be designed so that there is a degree of separation that will prevent any function or activity from having an adverse effect on the study.

1. **Animal care facilities**

   (a) A testing facility shall have a sufficient number of animal rooms or areas, as needed, to assure proper: (1) Separation of species or test systems, (2) isolation of individual projects, (3) quarantine of animals, and (4) routine or specialized housing of animals.

   (b) A testing facility shall have a number of animal rooms or areas separate to ensure isolation of studies being done with test systems or test and control articles known to be biohazardous, including volatile substances, aerosols, radioactive materials, and infectious agents.

   (c) Separate areas shall be provided, as appropriate, for the diagnosis, treatment, and control of laboratory animal diseases. These areas shall provide effective isolation for the housing of animals either known or suspected of being diseased, or of being carriers of disease, from other animals.

   (d) When animals are housed, facilities shall exist for the collection and disposal of all animal waste and refuse or for safe sanitary storage of waste before removal from the testing facility. Disposal facilities shall be so provided and operated as to minimize vermin infestation, odors, disease hazards, and environmental contamination.

2. **Animal supply facilities**

   There shall be storage areas, as needed, for feed, bedding, supplies, and equipment. Storage areas for feed and bedding shall be separated from areas housing the test systems and shall be protected against infestation or contamination. Perishable supplies shall be preserved by appropriate means.

3. **Facilities for handling test and control articles**

   (a) As necessary to prevent contamination or mix-ups, there shall be separate areas for:

      1. Receipt and storage of the test and control articles.
      2. Mixing of the test and control articles with a carrier, e.g., feed.
      3. Storage of the test and control article mixtures.

   (b) Storage areas for the test and/or control article and test and control mixtures shall be separate from areas housing the test systems and shall be adequate to preserve the identity, strength, purity, and stability of the articles and mixtures.

4. **Laboratory operation areas**

   Separate laboratory space shall be provided, as needed, for the performance of the routine and specialized procedures required by nonclinical laboratory studies.

5. **Specimen and data storage facilities**

   Space shall be provided for archives, limited to access by authorized personnel only, for the storage and retrieval of all raw data and specimens from completed studies.

Equipment

Equipment used in the generation, measurement, or assessment of data and equipment used for facility environmental control shall be of appropriate design and adequate capacity to function according to the protocol and shall be suitably located for operation, inspection, cleaning, and maintenance.

Maintenance and Calibration of Equipment

(a) Equipment shall be adequately inspected, cleaned, and maintained. Equipment used for the generation, measurement, or assessment of data shall be adequately tested, calibrated and/or standardized.

(b) The written standard operating procedures required shall set forth in sufficient detail the methods, materials, and schedules to be used in the routine inspection, cleaning, maintenance, testing, calibration, and/or standardization of equipment, and shall specify, when appropriate, remedial action to be taken in the event of failure or malfunction of equipment. The written standard operating procedures shall designate the person responsible for the performance of each operation.

(c) Written records shall be maintained of all inspection, maintenance, testing, calibrating and/or standardizing operations. These records, containing the date of the operation, shall describe whether the maintenance operations were routine and followed the written standard operating procedures. Written records shall be kept of non-routine repairs performed on equipment as a result of failure and malfunction. Such records shall document the nature of the defect, how and when the defect was discovered, and any remedial action taken in response to the defect.

Testing Facilities Operation

Standard operating procedures.

(a) A testing facility shall have standard operating procedures in writing setting forth nonclinical laboratory study methods that management is satisfied are adequate to ensure the quality and integrity of the data generated in the course of a study. All deviations in a study from standard operating procedures shall be authorized by the study director and shall be documented in the raw data. Significant changes in established standard operating procedures shall be properly authorized in writing by management.

(b) Standard operating procedures shall be established for, but not limited to, the following:

1. Animal room preparation.
2. Animal care.
3. Receipt, identification, storage, handling, mixing, and method of sampling of the test and control articles.
4. Test system observations.
5. Laboratory tests.
6. Handling of animals found moribund or dead during study.
7. Necropsy of animals or postmortem examination of animals.
8. Collection and identification of specimens.
9. Histopathology.
10. Data handling, storage, and retrieval.
11. Maintenance and calibration of equipment.
12. Transfer, proper placement, and identification of animals.

(c) Each laboratory area shall have immediately available laboratory manuals and standard operating procedures relative to the laboratory procedures being performed. Published literature may be used as a supplement to standard operating procedures.

(d) A historical file of standard operating procedures, and all revisions thereof, including the dates of such revisions, shall be maintained.

Reagents and Solutions

All reagents and solutions in the laboratory areas shall be labeled to indicate identity, titer or concentration, storage requirements, and expiration date. Deteriorated or outdated reagents and solutions shall not be used.

Animal Care

(a) There shall be standard operating procedures for the housing, feeding, handling, and care of animals.

(b) All newly received animals from outside sources shall be isolated and their health status shall be evaluated in accordance with acceptable veterinary medical practice.

(c) At the initiation of a nonclinical laboratory study, animals shall be free of any disease or condition that might interfere with the purpose or conduct of the study. If, during the course of the study, the animals' contract such a disease or condition, the diseased animals shall be isolated, if necessary. These animals may be treated for disease or signs of disease provided that such treatment does not interfere with the study. The diagnosis, authorizations of treatment, description of treatment, and each date of treatment shall be documented and shall be retained.

(d) Warm-blooded animals, excluding suckling rodents, used in laboratory procedures that require manipulations and observations over an extended period of time or in studies that require the animals to be removed from and returned to their home cages for any reason (e.g., cage cleaning, treatment, etc.), shall receive appropriate identification. All information needed to specifically identify each animal within an animal-housing unit shall appear on the outside of that unit.

(e) Animals of different species shall be housed in separate rooms when necessary. Animals of the same species, but used in different studies, should not ordinarily be housed in the same room when inadvertent exposure to control or test articles or animal mix-up could affect the outcome of either study. If such mixed housing is necessary, adequate differentiation by space and identification shall be made.

(f) Animal cages, racks and accessory equipment shall be cleaned and sanitized at appropriate intervals.

(g) Feed and water used for the animals shall be analyzed periodically to ensure that contaminants known to be capable of interfering with the study and reasonably expected to be present in such feed or water are not present at levels above those specified in the protocol. Documentation of such analyses shall be maintained as raw data.

(h) Bedding used in animal cages or pens shall not interfere with the purpose or conduct of the study and shall be changed as often as necessary to keep the animals dry and clean.

If any pest control materials are used, the use shall be documented. Cleaning and pest control materials that interfere with the study shall not be used.

Test and Control Articles

Test and control article characterization.

(a) The identity, strength, purity, and composition or other characteristics which will appropriately define the test or control article shall be determined for each batch and shall be documented. Methods of synthesis, fabrication, or derivation of the test and control articles shall be documented by the sponsor or the testing facility. In those cases where marketed products are used as control articles, such products will be characterized by their labeling.

(b) The stability of each test or control article shall be determined by the testing facility or by the sponsor either: (1) Before study initiation, or (2) concomitantly according to written standard operating procedures, which provide for periodic analysis of each batch.

(c) Each storage container for a test or control article shall be labeled by name, chemical abstract number or code number, batch number, expiration date, if any, and, where appropriate, storage conditions necessary to maintain the identity, strength, purity, and composition of the test or control article. Storage containers shall be assigned to a particular test article for the duration of the study.

(d) For studies of more than 4 weeks' duration, reserve samples from each batch of test and control articles shall be retained for the specified period of time.

Test and Control Article Handling

Procedures shall be established for a system for the handling of the test and control articles to ensure that:

(a) There is proper storage.

(b) Distribution is made in a manner designed to preclude the possibility of contamination, deterioration, or damage.

(c) Proper identification is maintained throughout the distribution process.

(d) The receipt and distribution of each batch is documented. Such documentation shall include the date and quantity of each batch distributed or returned.

Mixtures of articles with carriers.

(a) For each test or control article that is mixed with a carrier, tests by appropriate analytical methods shall be conducted:

1. To determine the uniformity of the mixture and to determine, periodically, the concentration of the test or control article in the mixture.
2. To determine the stability of the test and control articles in the mixture as required by the conditions of the study either:

   (i) Before study initiation, or

(ii) Concomitantly according to written standard operating procedures which provide for periodic analysis of the test and control articles in the mixture.

(b) Where any of the components of the test or control article carrier mixture has an expiration date, that date shall be clearly shown on the container. If more than one component has an expiration date, the earliest date shall be shown.

Protocol and Conduct of a Nonclinical Laboratory Study Protocol

(a) Each study shall have an approved written protocol that clearly indicates the objectives and all methods for the conduct of the study. The protocol shall contain, as applicable, the following information:

1. A descriptive title and statement of the purpose of the study.
2. Identification of the test and control articles by name, chemical abstract number, or code number.
3. The name of the sponsor and the name and address of the testing facility at which the study is being conducted.
4. The number, body weight range, sex, source of supply, species, strain, substrain, and age of the test system.
5. The procedure for identification of the test system.
6. A description of the experimental design, including the methods for the control of bias.
7. A description and/or identification of the diet used in the study as well as solvents, emulsifiers, and/or other materials used to solubilize or suspend the test or control articles before mixing with the carrier. The description shall include specifications for acceptable levels of contaminants that are reasonably expected to be present in the dietary materials and are known to be capable of interfering with the purpose or conduct of the study if present at levels greater than established by the specifications.
8. Each dosage level, expressed in milligrams per kilogram of body weight or other appropriate units, of the test or control article to be administered and the method and frequency of administration.
9. The type and frequency of tests, analyses, and measurements to be made.
10. The records to be maintained.

11. The date of approval of the protocol by the sponsor and the dated signature of the study director.
12. A statement of the proposed statistical methods to be used.

(b) All changes in or revisions of an approved protocol and the reasons therefore shall be documented, signed by the study director, dated, and maintained with the protocol.

Conduct of a Nonclinical Laboratory Study

(a) The nonclinical laboratory study shall be conducted in accordance with the protocol.
(b) The test systems shall be monitored in conformity with the protocol.
(c) Specimens shall be identified by test system, study, nature, and date of collection. This information shall be located on the specimen container or shall accompany the specimen in a manner that precludes error in the recording and storage of data.
(d) Records of gross findings for a specimen from postmortem observations should be available to a pathologist when examining that specimen histopathologically.
(e) All data generated during the conduct of a nonclinical laboratory study, except those that are generated by automated data collection systems, shall be recorded directly, promptly, and legibly in ink. All data entries shall be dated on the date of entry and signed or initialed by the person entering the data. Any change in entries shall be made so as not to obscure the original entry, shall indicate the reason for such change, and shall be dated and signed or identified at the time of the change. In automated data collection systems, the individual responsible for direct data input shall be identified at the time of data input. Any change in automated data entries shall be made so as not to obscure the original entry, shall indicate the reason for change, shall be dated, and the responsible individual shall be identified.

Records and Reports

Reporting of nonclinical laboratory study results.

(a) A final report shall be prepared for each nonclinical laboratory study and shall include, but not necessarily be limited to, the following:
    1. Name and address of the facility performing the study and the dates on which the study was initiated and completed.
    2. Objectives and procedures stated in the approved protocol, including any changes in the original protocol.
    3. Statistical methods employed for analyzing the data.

4. The test and control articles identified by name, chemical abstracts number or code number, strength, purity, and composition or other appropriate characteristics.
5. Stability of the test and control articles under the conditions of administration.
6. A description of the methods used.
7. A description of the test system used. Where applicable, the final report shall include the number of animals used, sex, body weight range, source of supply, species, strain and substrain, age, and procedure used for identification.
8. A description of the dosage, dosage regimen, route of administration, and duration.
9. A description of all circumstances that may have affected the quality or integrity of the data.
10. The name of the study director, the names of other scientists or professionals, and the names of all supervisory personnel, involved in the study.
11. A description of the transformations, calculations, or operations performed on the data, a summary and analysis of the data, and a statement of the conclusions drawn from the analysis.
12. The signed and dated reports of each of the individual scientists or other professionals involved in the study.
13. The locations where all specimens, raw data, and the final report are to be stored.
14. The statement prepared and signed by the quality assurance unit

(b) The final report shall be signed and dated by the study director.

(c) Corrections or additions to a final report shall be in the form of an amendment by the study director. The amendment shall clearly identify that part of the final report that is being added to or corrected and the reasons for the correction or addition and shall be signed and dated by the person responsible.

Disqualification of Testing Facilities

Purpose

(a) The purposes of disqualification are:

1. To permit the exclusion from consideration of completed studies that were conducted by a testing facility which has failed to comply with the requirements of the good laboratory practice regulations until it can be adequately demonstrated that such noncompliance did not occur during, or did not affect the validity or acceptability of data generated by, a particular study; and

2. To exclude from consideration all studies completed after the date of disqualification until the facility can satisfy the Commissioner that it will conduct studies in compliance with such regulations.

(b) The determination that a nonclinical laboratory study may not be considered in support of an application for a research or marketing permit does not, however, relieve the applicant for such a permit of any obligation under any other applicable regulation to submit the results of the study to the Food and Drug Administration.

Grounds for Disqualification

The Commissioner may disqualify a testing facility upon finding all of the following:

(a) The testing facility failed to comply with one or more of the regulations set forth in this part (or any other regulations regarding such facilities in this chapter);

(b) The noncompliance adversely affected the validity of the nonclinical laboratory studies; and

(c) Other lesser regulatory actions (e.g., warnings or rejection of individual studies) have not been or will probably not be adequate to achieve compliance with the good laboratory practice regulations.

Notice of and opportunity for hearing on proposed disqualification

(a) Whenever the Commissioner has information indicating that grounds exist under the guideline which in his opinion justify disqualification of a testing facility, he may issue to the testing facility a written notice proposing that the facility be disqualified.

(b) A hearing on the disqualification shall be conducted in accordance with the requirements for a regulatory hearing set forth in the guidelines.

Final Order on Disqualification

(a) If the Commissioner, after the regulatory hearing, or after the time for requesting a hearing expires without a request being made, upon an evaluation of the administrative record of the disqualification proceeding, makes the findings required in the guidelines, he shall issue a final order disqualifying the facility. Such order shall include a statement of the basis for that determination. Upon issuing a final order, the Commissioner shall notify (with a copy of the order) the testing facility of the action.

(b) If the Commissioner, after a regulatory hearing or after the time for requesting a hearing expires without a request being made, upon an evaluation of the administrative record of the disqualification proceeding, does not make the findings required in the guidelines, he shall issue a final order terminating the disqualification proceeding. Such order shall include a statement of the basis for that determination. Upon issuing a final order the Commissioner shall notify the testing facility and provide a copy of the order.

Actions upon Disqualification

(a) Once a testing facility has been disqualified, each application for a research or marketing permit, whether approved or not, containing or relying upon any nonclinical laboratory study conducted by the disqualified testing facility may be examined to determine whether such study was or would be essential to a decision. If it is determined that a study was or would be essential, the Food and Drug Administration shall also determine whether the study is acceptable, notwithstanding the disqualification of the facility. Any study done by a testing facility before or after disqualification may be presumed to be unacceptable, and the person relying on the study may be required to establish that the study was not affected by the circumstances that led to the disqualification, e.g., by submitting validating information. If the study is then determined to be unacceptable, such data will be eliminated from consideration in support of the application; and such elimination may serve as new information justifying the termination or withdrawal of approval of the application.

(b) No nonclinical laboratory study begun by a testing facility after the date of the facility's disqualification shall be considered in support of any application for a research or marketing permit, unless the facility has been reinstated under the guidelines. The determination that a study may not be considered in support of an application for a research or marketing permit does not, however, relieve the applicant for such a permit of any obligation under any other applicable regulation to submit the results of the study to the Food and Drug Administration.

Public Disclosure of Information Regarding Disqualification

(a) Upon issuance of a final order disqualifying a testing facility under the guidelines, the Commissioner may notify all or any interested persons. Such notice may be given at the discretion of the Commissioner whenever he believes that such disclosure would further the public interest or would promote compliance with the good laboratory practice regulations set forth in this regulation. Such notice, if given, shall include a copy of the final order issued under the guideline and shall state that the disqualification constitutes a determination by the Food and Drug Administration that nonclinical laboratory studies performed by the facility will not be considered by the Food and Drug Administration in support of any application for a research or marketing permit. If such notice is sent to another Federal Government agency, the Food and Drug Administration will recommend that the agency also consider whether or not it should accept nonclinical laboratory studies performed by the testing facility. If such notice is sent to any other person, it shall state that it is given because of the relationship between the testing facility and the person being notified and that the Food and Drug Administration is not advising or recommending that any action be taken by the person notified.

(b) A determination that a testing facility has been disqualified and the administrative record regarding such determination are disclosable to the public under the guidelines.

Alternative or Additional Actions to Disqualification

(a) Disqualification of a testing facility under this subpart is independent of, and neither in lieu of nor a precondition to, other proceedings or actions authorized by the act. The Food and Drug Administration may, at any time, institute against a testing facility and/or against the sponsor of a nonclinical laboratory study that has been submitted to the Food and Drug Administration any appropriate judicial proceedings (civil or criminal) and any other appropriate regulatory action, in addition to or in lieu of, and prior to, simultaneously with, or subsequent to, disqualification. The Food and Drug Administration may also refer the matter to another Federal, State, or local government law enforcement or regulatory agency for such action as that agency deems appropriate.

(b) The Food and Drug Administration may refuse to consider any particular nonclinical laboratory study in support of an application for a research or marketing permit, if it finds that the study was not conducted in accordance with the good laboratory practice regulations set forth in this guidelines, without disqualifying the testing facility that conducted the study or undertaking other regulatory action.

Suspension or Termination of a Testing Facility by a Sponsor

Termination of a testing facility by a sponsor is independent of, and neither in lieu of nor a precondition to, proceedings or actions authorized by this subpart. If a sponsor terminates or suspends a testing facility from further participation in a nonclinical laboratory study that is being conducted as part of any application for a research or marketing permit that has been submitted to any Center of the Food and Drug Administration (whether approved or not), it shall notify that Center in writing within 15 working days of the action; the notice shall include a statement of the reasons for such action. Suspension or termination of a testing facility by a sponsor does not relieve it of any obligation under any other applicable regulation to submit the results of the study to the Food and Drug Administration.

Reinstatement of a Disqualified Testing Facility

A testing facility that has been disqualified may be reinstated as an acceptable source of nonclinical laboratory studies to be submitted to the Food and Drug Administration if the Commissioner determines, upon an evaluation of the submission of the testing facility, that the facility can adequately assure that it will conduct future nonclinical laboratory studies in compliance with the good laboratory practice regulations set forth in this part and, if any studies are currently being conducted, that the quality and integrity of such studies have not been seriously compromised. A disqualified testing facility that wishes to be so reinstated shall present in writing to the Commissioner reasons why it believes it should be reinstated and a detailed description of the corrective actions it has taken or intends to take to assure that the acts or omissions which led to its disqualification will not recur. The Commissioner may condition reinstatement upon the testing facility being found in compliance with the good laboratory practice regulations upon an inspection. If a testing facility is reinstated, the Commissioner shall so notify the testing facility and all organizations and persons who were notified, under guideline of the disqualification of the testing facility. A determination that a testing facility has been reinstated is disclosable to the public under this guideline.

CHPATER - 14

Calibration and Validation of Analytical Instruments

Learning Objectives

To learn about

- Calibration and Qualification - Definitions and Principles
- Validation - Definitions, Importance and scope
- Types of validation,
- Validation Master Plan
- Calibration of UV-Visible Spectrophotometer
- Calibration of IR Spectrophotometer
- Calibration of Spectrofluorometer
- Calibration of HPLC System
- Calibration of HPTLC
- Calibration of Gas Chromatography
- Calibration of Ph meter
- Calibration of Balance
- Principles of Analytical Method Validation (System Suitability, Specificity, Linearity,
- Range, Accuracy, Precision, LOD, LOQ, Robustness, Forced Degradation Study)

Introduction

Analytical instruments are used for a specific analysis of drugs and pharmaceuticals. Regular performance verification of analytical instruments is made to ensure that they are working as expected to serve the purpose. The analytical instruments should be properly validated and calibrated to demonstrate that they are suitable for their intended purpose.

Calibration

Calibration is a process which ensures the reading on an instrument is accurate with reference to established standards. Calibration is performed using primary reference standards. Instruments need to be calibrated before using.

Need for Calibration

Calibration is needed in the following situations:

(i) With a new instrument.
(ii) When a specified time period is elapsed.
(iii) When a specified usage (operating hours) has elapsed.
(iv) When an instrument has had a shock or vibration which potentially may have put it out of calibration.
(v) Sudden changes in weather.
(vi) Whenever observations appear questionable.

Validation

Validation is a detailed process of confirming that the instrument is installed correctly, that it is operating effectively, and that it is performing without error. Validation is divided into the following subsections:

(i) Cleaning validation
(ii) Process validation
(iii) Analytical method validation
(iv) Computer system validation

Calibration of UV-VIS spectrophotometer

The UV-Visible spectrophotometer is calibrated based on the following parameters

(i) Wavelength accuracy
(ii) Stray light
(iii) Resolution
(iv) Photometric accuracy
(v) Noise
(vi) Baseline flatness
(vii) Stability

Wavelength Accuracy

It is defined as the deviation of the wavelength reading at an absorption band or emission band from the wavelength of the band.

Test

Wavelength accuracy verification is checked by comparing the recorded wavelength of the peak against the value of reference standard. Commonly used wavelength standards include ¬Deuterium lamp,

- Mercury vapor lamp,
- Holmium oxide filter, and
- Holmium oxide solution (4% holmium oxide in 10% perchloric acid in a 1-cm cell)

Acceptance ±1 nm in the UV range (200 to 380 nm) and ±3 nm in the visible range (380 to 800 nm). Three repeated scans of the same peak should be within ±0.5 nm.

Stray light

Stray light is defined as the detected light of any wavelength that is outside the bandwidth of the wavelength selected. Test: - Three test solutions prepared and measured the stray light at 200 nm, 220 nm and 340 nm Acceptance: - The transmittance of the solution in a 1 cm cell should be less than 0.01 or the absorbance value should be greater than 2.

At 1% transmittance, stray light at 1% of the incident light intensity can cause a 15% drop in absorbance

Resolution power

The resolution of a UV-VIS spectrophotometer is related to its spectral bandwidth (SBW). The smaller the spectral width, the finer the resolution. The SBW depends on the slit width and the dispersive power of the monochromator

Test

0.02%v/v toluene in hexane is used to test the resolution power of the spectrophotometer. The absorbance measured at 269 nm and 266 nm. Acceptance: - The ratio of the absorbance at 269 nm and absorbance at 266 nm should be greater than 1.5

Noise

Noise in the measurement affects the accuracy at both ends of the absorbance scale. Photon noise from the light source affects the accuracy of the measurements leads to low absorbance.

Test

Air is scanned in the absorbance mode for 10 min. Peak to noise is recorded at 500nm. Root mean square noise is then calculated.

Acceptance: The RMS noise should be less than 0.001 AU

Baseline flatness

The flat baseline test demonstrates the ability of the instrument to normalize the light intensity measurement and the spectral output at different wavelengths throughout the spectral range.

Test

Air is scanned in the absorbance mode. The highest and lowest deflections in the absorbance unit are recorded.

Acceptance

The deflection is typically less than 0.01AU

Stability

The lamp intensity is a function of the age of the lamp, temperature fluctuation, and wavelength of the measurement. These changes can lead to errors in the value of the measurements, over an extended period of time.

Test

Air is scanned in the absorbance mode for 60 min at specific wavelength (340nm). The highest and lowest deflections in the absorbance unit are recorded.

Acceptance

The deflection is less than 0.002 AU/h

Photometric accuracy

Photometric accuracy is determined by comparing the difference between the measured absorbance of the reference materials and the established value.

Test

Either neutral density filters or potassium dichromate solutions are used.

Acceptance

Six replicate measurements of the 0.006%w/v potassium dichromate solution at 235, 257, 313 and 350 nm should be less than 0.5% RSD.

Linearity

The linear dynamic range of the measurement is limited by stray light at high absorbance and by noise at low absorbance. The accuracy of the quantification of the sample depends on the precision and linearity of the measurements.

Test

A series of Potassium dichromate solution of concentration 20, 40, 60, 80 and 100mg/L in 0.005M sulfuric acid. The absorptions of various wavelengths are plotted against the concentration of the solution and the correlation coefficients are calculated. Acceptance: - Correlation coefficient $r \geq 0.999$

Calibration of IR Spectrophotometer

Calibration of IR spectrophotometer is based on the following parameters

(i) Wave number verification

(ii) Resolution performance

Wave number verification

Prepare polystyrene film with thickness 0.04 mm and verify the wavenumber Observed wavenumber Minimum tolerance Maximum tolerance 3058.5 3061.5 2848.0 2851.0 1941.4 1944.4 1600.2 1602.2 1582.0 1584.0 1153.5 1155.5 1027.3 1029.3

Resolution performance

Difference between %T at 2851 cm -1 and 2870 cm -1 Difference between %T at 1583 cm -1 and 1589 cm -1 Limit NLT 18% NLT 12% Actual

Calibration of Spectrofluorimeter

Calibration of spectrofluorimeter is based on the following parameters

(i) Sensitivity of the instrument checked by using primary standard

(ii) Prepare 1ppm solution of quinine sulphate solution in 0.1M sulphuric acid.

(iii) Primary wavelength set at 366 nm and check the sensitivity of the instrument.

Calibration of HPLC

Calibration of HPLC is based on the following parameters

(i) Flow rate accuracy

(ii) Injector accuracy

(iii) System precision

(iv) Wavelength accuracy

(v) Detector linearity

(vi) Injector linearity

(vii) Gradient performance check

(viii) Column oven temperature accuracy

Flow Rate Accuracy

The performance of pump module is the ability to maintain accurate and consistent flow of the mobile phase. Poor flow rate will affect the retention time and resolution of the separation.

Test

The flow rate accuracy at 2 mL/min can be verified by using a calibrated stopwatch to measure the time it takes to collect 25 mL of effluent from the pump into a 25 mL volumetric flask. **Acceptance: -** ±2.0% 0f the set flow rate

Gradient accuracy

The accuracy and linearity of the gradient solvent delivery can be verified indirectly by monitoring the absorbance change when the composition of the two solvents from two different channels changes.

Test

Channel A is filled with a pure solvent such as methanol and Channel B is filled with a solvent containing a UV-active tracer such as caffeine (ca. 15 mg per litre of solvent).

The gradient profile is programmed to vary the composition of the mixture from 100% A to 100% B in a short period of time, and then changed back to 100% A in a stepwise manner. If the composition of the 20% A and 80% B mixture is accurate, the height B1, which corresponds to the absorbance at 80% B The linearity of the gradient delivery can be verified by plotting the absorbance at various mobile-phase composition versus sample compositions.

System precision

Weigh accurately 60 mg of caffeine into 100 mL volumetric flask. Dissolve and dilute to the volume with mobile phase. Transfer 10 mL of this solution into 100 mL flask and make up with mobile phase. Inject blank followed by standard preparation in 6 replicates. Note down the areas and retention times.

Acceptance

The % RSD of retention time and peak area should be <1.0%

Wavelength accuracy

Inject blank followed by standard preparation and note down the height or absorbance.

Acceptance

The maximum absorbance should be ± 2 nm.

Detector linearity

The linearity of the detector response can be checked by pumping or by filling the flow cell with a series of standard solution of various concentration. Aqueous caffeine solutions are convenient for the linearity measurement. The correlation coefficient between sample concentration and response can be calculated to determine the linearity.

Acceptance

$R \geq 0.999$

Injector linearity

Linearity is important for methods that require the use of variable injection volumes. The linearity of the injector can be demonstrated by making injections, typically 5,10,20,50 and 100 μL to cover the range 0 to 100 μL. The response of the injection is plotted against the injection volume. The correlation coefficient of the plot is used in evaluation of the injector linearity.

Acceptance

$R \geq 0.999$

Column oven temperature accuracy

- The efficiency of HPLC column varies with column temperature.
- The temperature accuracy of the column heater is evaluated by placing a calibrated thermometer in the column compartment to measure the actual compartment temperature.
- The thermometer readings are compared to the preset temperature at 40 and 60°C.

Acceptance

The resulting oven temperature from the thermometer display should be within ± 2°C of the set temperature.

Calibration of HPTLC

Calibration of HPTLC is based on the following parameters

Spotting & Detection capacity

Requirements

Alumina glass plates Sodium salicylate 96%v/v alcohol

Preparation of stock solution

Stock solution-1 Weigh 500 mg of sodium salicylate in 250 mL volumetric flask dissolve and dilute with 96%v/v alcohol.

Stock solution-2 100 mg of sod. salicylate in 250 mL volumetric flask, dissolve and dilute with 96% v/v alcohol.

Procedure

Spot 5μL of each solution observe at 254 nm, 366 nm.

Acceptance

The spots shall be comparable intensity wise. Spot due to stock solution-2 shall be visible at 254 nm. Spot due to stock solution-1 shall be visible at 366 nm.

Calibration of Gas Chromatography

Calibration of Gas chromatography is based on the following parameters

(i) Flow rate accuracy
(ii) Column oven temperature accuracy
(iii) System precision
(iv) System precision for head space auto sampler
(v) Detector linearity
(vi) Detector noise and drift test

Flow rate accuracy

Connect the digital flow meter to the detector outlet port.

- Set the carrier gas flow and wait till it reaches the set flow.
- Note the observed flow in replicate.
- Repeat the procedure for other carrier gases such as Hydrogen and Air.

Acceptance

The flow rate of carrier gas should be ±10% of set flow.

Column oven temperature accuracy

Place the thermometer in the column oven and set the column oven temperature at 40°C. Wait till the temperature stabilizes. Note the observed temperature over a period of 10 mts. Repeat the procedure for 100°C, 150°C and 190°C.

Acceptance

The resulting oven temperature from the thermometer display should be within ±2°C of the set temperature.

System precision

Transfer 20 mL of methanol, Ethanol and acetone into 100 mL volumetric flask and make up with ethyl acetate. Inject blank followed by standard preparation in 6 replicates. Note down the areas and retention times.

Acceptance

The %RSD of retention time should be not more than 1.0% & peak area NMT 5.0%.

System precision for head space auto sampler

Prepare a standard mixture solution Methylene dichloride (0.6g), Chloroform (0.06g), Trichloroethane (0.08g),1, 4, Dioxane 0.38g) in 50 mL volumetric flask containing 40 mL of Dimethyl formamide.

- Finally make up to the volume with DMF(Solution-A).
- Take 0.5 mL of standard solution A in 6 different vials and seal caps and crimp.
- Place these vials on head space sampler. Prepare a blank vial also.
- Load the vials in head space sampler tray.
- Blank vials followed by the standard vials.

Acceptance

The %RSD of retention time should be NMT 1.0% and Peak area should b NMT 15.0%

Detector linearity Detector linearity solutions 10 mL of Methanol, Ethanol, Acetone make up to 100 mL with Ethyl acetate 15mL of Methanol, Ethanol, Acetone make up to 100 mL with Ethyl acetate 20mL of Methanol, Ethanol, Acetone make up to 100 mL with Ethyl acetate 25mL of Methanol, Ethanol, Acetone make up to 100 mL with Ethyl acetate 30 mL of Methanol, Ethanol, Acetone make up to 100 mL with Ethyl acetate Solution A Solution B Solution C Solution D Solution E

Procedure

Inject blank, followed by detector linearity solutions and record the peak responses. Draw a standard plot between the concentration Vs the peak responses. Acceptance The plot should be linear and regression coefficient should NLT 0.99

Detector noise and drift test

After GC is ready run the system up to 15mts through single run. After completion of run calculate noise and drift through software. Acceptance Noise NMT 100 μV Drift NMT 2500μV/hr

Schedule for calibration of major instruments INSTRUMENT INTERVAL (MONTHS)

- HPLC 3 ± 7 days
- Gas chromatography 3 ± 7 days
- UV-Visible spectrophotometer Monthly once ± 3 days
- IR spectrophotometer Monthly once ± 3 days
- NMR spectrophotometer 6 ± 15 days
- Flourimeter 3 ± 7 days
- pH meter Daily Analytical Balance Daily

Calibration of pH Meters with pH 7 and pH 2 Buffers

1. Select the pH Mode and set the temperature control knob to 25°C. Adjust the cal 2 knob to read 100%.
2. Rinse the electrode with deionized water and blot dry using a piece of tissue (Shurwipes or Kimwipes are available in the labs).
3. Place the electrode in the solution of pH 7 buffer, allow the display to stabilize and, then, set the display to read 7 by adjusting cal 1. Remove the electrode from the buffer.
4. Rinse the electrode with deionized water and blot dry using a piece of tissue (Shurwipes or Kimwipes are available in the labs).
5. Place the electrode in the solution of pH 2 buffer, allow the display to stabilize and, then, set the display to read 2 by adjusting cal 2. Remove the electrode from the buffer.
6. Rinse the electrode with deionized water and blot dry using a piece of tissue (Shurwipes or Kimwipes, as before).

NOTE: Buffer solution is made available in individually labelled 2 oz. bottles.

The buffers are to be used in these containers, only

Do not pour them into other containers at any time.

After use, cap the bottles so that the buffers can be re-used.

Measuring pH

1. Make sure that the meter is set to the pH Mode and adjust the temperature to 25°C.
2. Place the electrode in the sample to be tested.
3. The pH of the solution appears in the display.
   NOTE: Allow the display to stabilize before taking reading
4. Rinse the pH electrode and place it back in the storage solution.

Calibration of Balance

Standard operating procedure to evaluate the performance of Analytical Balance used for the analysis in pharmaceutical quality control by accuracy and precision tests.

Procedure

(i) Operate the instrument as per respective Standard Operating Procedure.

(ii) Switch 'ON' the instrument.

(iii) Switch 'ON' the balance.

(iv) The display will blink with 8.8.8.8.8.8.

(v) After few seconds, the display will show 0.00 g.

(vi) If display is not stable, press the TARE key & wait till the display shows 0.00 g.

For Accuracy

(i) Place 5 gm. on the weighing pan.

(ii) Note the weight.

(iii) Calculate the difference between the weight in certificate and observed weight.

(iv) Repeat the above steps using 50gm & 100 gm. weights.

For precision

(i) Place 5 gm. in the weighing pan.

(ii) Note the weight.

(iii) Repeat the above two steps nine times.

(iv) Calculate the Standard deviation.

(v) Calculate the measurement uncertainty using following equation.

$$\text{Measurement uncertainty} = \frac{2 \times \text{SD}}{\text{Actual weight from certificate}}$$

Frequency

(i) Internal calibration and accuracy = Daily

(ii) Precision: Once in a month

General Principles of Analytical Method Validation

The analytical method should give accurate and reliable results for the purpose for which it is used. Validation is a topic of current interest in pharmaceutical manufacturing, quality control and quality Assurance. In simple terms validation means testing and conforming or proving with appropriate documentation that an equipment, a process and a method is working as expected. The main objective of validation of an analytical procedure is to demonstrate that the procedure is suitable for its intended purpose. The process of validation of analytical method is adopted to confirm that the employed analytical procedure for a specific test meet the intended requirements. Guidelines from the USP, ICH, FDA etc., can provide a framework for validations of analytical methods.(1-4) Results from the method validation can be considered to judge its quality, reliability as well consistency pertaining to analytical results. ICH guidelines Q2(R1) provides the validation parameters of analytical methods and their specifications. The essential guidelines under Q2(R1) are as follows.

System Suitability

System suitability testing is to decide whether a chromatographic system is suitable for being used in day today routine analysis.

The parameters used in the system suitability tests include:

1. Number of theoretical plates or Efficiency (N).
2. Capacity factor (K).
3. Separation or Relative retention (α).
4. Resolution (Rs).
5. Tailing factor (T).
6. Relative Standard Deviation (RSD).

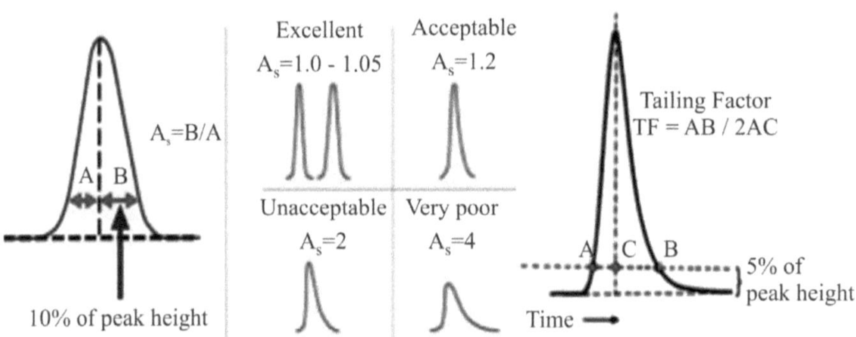

Table 14.1 Acceptance criteria for system suitability parameters

S. No	Parameter	Acceptance criteria
1	Number of theoretical plates or Efficiency (N)	> 2000
2	Capacity factor (K)	< 1
3	Separation or Relative retention (α)	> 1
4	Resolution (Rs)	> 1.5
5	Tailing factor or Asymmetry(T)	< 2
6	Relative Standard Deviation (RSD)	< 2

The acceptance criteria for system suitability parameters are given in Table 14.1

Specificity

Specificity is the ability to assess unequivocally the analyte in the presence of other compounds that may be likely to be present. It is not always possible to demonstrate that an analytical procedure is specific for a particular analyte (complete discrimination). In this case a combination of two or more analytical procedures is recommended to achieve the necessary level of discrimination.

Forced Degradation Studies

Forced degradation is undertaken to demonstrate specificity when developing stability indicating method. A stability indicating method is one that accurately quantitates the active ingredient without interference from degradation products, excipients and other potential impurities.

Linearity

A linear relationship should be evaluated across the range (see section 3) of the analytical procedure. It may be demonstrated directly on the active substance (by dilution of a standard stock solution) and/or on separate weighing of synthetic mixtures of the product components, using the proposed procedure.

Linearity should be evaluated by visual inspection of a plot of signals as a function of analyte concentration or content. test results should be evaluated by appropriate statistical methods, for example, by calculation of a regression line by the method of least squares.

Range

The specified range is normally derived from linearity studies and depends on the intended application of the procedure. The following minimum specified ranges should be considered

- For the assay of an active substance or a finished product: normally from 80 to 120 percent of the test concentration.
- For content uniformity, covering a minimum of 70 to 130 percent of the test concentration.
- For dissolution testing: +/-20 % over the specified range; e.g., if the specifications for a controlled released product cover a region from 20%, after 1 hour, up to 90%, after 24 hours, the validated range would be 0-110% of the label claim.
- For the determination of an impurity: from the reporting level of an impurity1 to 120% of the specification

Accuracy

The accuracy of a measurement is defined as the closeness of the measured value to the true value. In a method with high accuracy, a sample (whose "true value" is known) is analyzed and the measured value is identical to the true value. Typically, accuracy is represented and determined by recovery studies. There are three ways to determine accuracy:

1. Comparison to a reference standard.
2. Recovery of the analyte spiked into blank matrix.
3. Standard addition of the analyte.

Assay

Active Substance

(a) Application of an analytical procedure to an analyte of known purity (e.g. reference material).

(b) Comparison of the results of the proposed analytical procedure with those of a second well-characterised procedure, the accuracy of which is stated and/or defined (independent procedure).

(c) Accuracy may be inferred once precision, linearity and specificity have been established.

Impurities (Quantitation) Accuracy should be assessed on samples (substance/ product) spiked with known amounts of impurities.

Precision

Precision may be defined as the concordance of a series of measurements (n) of the same quantity. Precision expresses the „reproducibility" of a measurement.

Repeatability should be assessed using: (a) a minimum of 9 determinations covering the specified range for the procedure (e.g. 3 concentrations / 3 replicates each) or (a) a minimum of 6 determinations at 100% of the test concentration.

Intermediate Precision: The extent to which intermediate precision should be established depends on the circumstances under which the procedure is intended to be used.

Typical variations to be studied include days, analysts, equipment, etc. It is not considered necessary to study these effects individually. The use of an experimental design (matrix) is encouraged.

Reproducibility: Reproducibility is assessed by means of an inter-laboratory trial.

Detection Limit

LOQ is determined by the analysis of samples with known concentration of analyte and by establishing that minimum level at which the analyte can reliably detected, but not necessarily quantitated as precise value, under the stated experimental conditions. The detection limit is generally expressed in the concentration of analyte (ppm) in the sample.

Based on visual evaluation Visual evaluation may be used for non-instrumental methods but may also be used with instrumental methods. The detection limit is determined by the analysis of samples with known concentrations of analyte and by establishing the minimum level at which the analyte can be reliably detected.

Based on signal-to-noise This approach can only be applied to analytical procedures which exhibit baseline noise. Determination of the signal-to-noise ratio is performed by comparing measured signals from samples with known low concentrations of analyte with those of blank samples and establishing the minimum concentration at which the analyte can be reliably detected. A signal-to-noise ratio between 3 or 2:1 is generally considered acceptable for estimating the detection limit.

Based on the Standard Deviation of the Response and the Slope

The detection limit (DL) may be expressed as:

$$DL = 3.3\ \sigma\ S$$

where σ = the standard deviation of the response, S = the slope of the calibration curve

The slope S may be estimated from the calibration curve of the analyte. The estimate of σ may be carried out in a variety of ways, for example:

Based on the Standard Deviation of the Blank

Measurement of the magnitude of analytical background response is performed by analysing an appropriate number of blank samples and calculating the standard deviation of these responses.

Based on the Calibration Curve

A specific calibration curve should be studied using samples containing an analyte in the range of DL. The residual standard deviation of a regression line or the standard deviation of y-intercepts of regression lines may be used as the standard deviation.

Limit of Quantitation

Limit of quantitation is the least concentration of drug in a sample which is estimated with appropriate precision and accuracy under the affirmed experimental conditions.

Based on Visual Evaluation Visual evaluation may be used for non-instrumental methods but may also be used with instrumental methods. The quantitation limit is generally determined by the analysis of samples with known concentrations of analyte and by establishing the minimum level at which the analyte can be quantified with acceptable accuracy and precision.

Based on Signal-to-Noise Approach This approach can only be applied to analytical procedures that exhibit baseline noise. Determination of the signal-to-noise ratio is performed by comparing measured signals from samples with known low concentrations of analyte with those of blank samples and by establishing the minimum concentration at which the analyte can be reliably quantified. A typical signal-to-noise ratio is 10:1.

Based on the Standard Deviation of the Response and the Slope

The quantitation limit (QL) may be expressed as:

$$QL = 10\,\sigma\,S$$

Where, σ = the standard deviation of the response, S = the slope of the calibration curve

The slope S may be estimated from the calibration curve of the analyte. The estimate of σ may be carried out in a variety of ways including:

Based on Standard Deviation of the Blank

Measurement of the magnitude of analytical background response is performed by analysing an appropriate number of blank samples and calculating the standard deviation of these responses.

Based on the Calibration Curve

A specific calibration curve should be studied using samples, containing an analyte in the range of QL. The residual standard deviation of a regression line or the standard deviation of y-intercepts of regression lines may be used as the standard deviation.

Robustness

It should show the reliability of an analysis with respect to deliberate variations in method parameters.

Examples of typical variations are:

- Stability of analytical solutions,
- Extraction time in the case of liquid chromatography,
- Influence of variations of pH in a mobile phase,
- Influence of variations in mobile phase composition,
- Different columns (different lots and/or suppliers),
- Temperature.

CHPATER - **15**

Warehousing and Materials Management

Learning Objectives

To learn about

- Warehousing
- Functions and Benefits of Ware Housing
- Types of Warehouses
- Good Warehousing Practices of Pharmaceuticals
- cGMPs related to Warehousing
- Kanban Logistics for Pharmaceutical Warehousing
- Materials Management- Definition and Explanation
- Functions of Materials Management
- The objectives of materials management
- Advantages or benefits of materials management
- Challenges of material management:
- Organization of material management:
- Purchasing- Definition, Importance and objectives of purchasing
- Purchasing cycle
- Vendor rating
- Ethics in purchasing
- Value analysis
- Inventory Management
- Objectives of Inventory
- Benefits of Inventory management

Warehousing

Warehousing refers to the activities involving storage of goods on a large-scale in a systematic and orderly manner and making them available conveniently when needed. It involves holding or preserving goods in huge quantities from the time of their purchase or production till their actual use or sale. It creates time utility by bridging the time gap between production and consumption of goods. Materials which need warehousing include raw materials, consumable stores and spares, ready-made components and finished goods.

Characteristics of an Ideal Warehouse include convenient location; availability of mechanical appliances to load and unload goods; adequate space; cold storage facilities; proper arrangement for protection; sufficient parking space; round the clock security arrangement and latest fire fighting equipments

The following are the functions of ware house

- Storage of Goods
- Protection of Goods
- Risk Bearing
- Identification of Goods
- Financing
- Processing

Benefits of Ware Housing

1. Maximum usage of available floor space and building height
2. Increase storage capacity
3. High productivity
4. Operate faster and no delays
5. Efficient flow of materials
6. Provide buffer storage functions ‘
7. Ongoing operating costs eliminated

Types of Warehouses

1. Private Warehouses

These are operated by a company for shipping and storing its own products.

Owned and managed by manufacturers or traders. Farmers construct near their fields and wholesalers and retailers near their business centers and manufacturers near their factories.

Advantages of Private Warehouses:

- Better control over movement and storage
- Chances of errors and mistakes are less as products are handled by its own employees who have full knowledge
- Designing is done according to suitability of owner

- Greater flexibility with respect to storage and material handling needs

2. **Public or Government Warehouses**

   These provide storage and physical distribution services on rental basis. These are used by small firms and large firms. These provide storage facilities to traders, manufacturers, agriculturists against storage charge licensed by govt. These are licensed by government's example Central Warehousing Corporation, State Warehousing Corporation and Food Corporation of India.

   Advantages of Public Warehousing

   - More efficient and less expensive
   - Cost easily and exactly ascertained
   - Fixed cost distributed among many users
   - Strategically located and immediately available
   - Flexible to meet space requirements of different users
   - Companies have a wide choice of locations and warehouse types

3. **Co-Operative Warehouses**

   These are owned, Managed and Controlled by Co-operative societies. Facilities at most economical rates to members. Available widely in Punjab, Karnataka, Maharashtra and Andhra.

4. **Bonded Warehouses**

   These are licensed to accept imported goods for storage before payment of customs duty.

   Imported merchandise is stored and released only after payment of appropriate taxes.

   These are owned and operated by Port Trusts.

5. **Distribution Centers Or Warehouses**

   Designed to move goods. Large and highly automated. Receive goods from various plants and suppliers, take orders, fill them efficiently deliver to customers quickly. Located near the market owned or leased by manufacturers. Access to transport networks

6. **Cold Storage**

   Preserve perishability of goods against payment of a storage charge. Temperature variation is controlled to degree necessary for certain sensitive items

7. **Export and Import Warehouses**

   These are located near ports where international trade is undertaken. These provide storage facilities for goods awaiting onward movements.

8. **Climate-Controlled Warehouse**

   These provide storage of many products which need special handling conditions .Freezers for frozen products, humidity controlled environment for delicate products, produce or flowers etc.

Good Warehousing Practices of Pharmaceuticals

Pharmaceuticals are stringently regulated by the Food and Drug Administration (FDA). The FDA's regulatory standards for the industry are referred to as Current Good Manufacturing Practice (CGMPs; also known as "Good Manufacturing Practice" [GMP]) standards. These standards apply to **warehouses,** processes, and to the drugs themselves.

cGMPs Related to Warehousing

These include the following

1. Drugs must be stored to prevent contamination, and be positioned to allow for inspection and cleaning of the area.
2. Each lot of drug products must be identified with a distinctive (and traceable) code, and the lot's status must be identified (approved, quarantined, and rejected).
3. Written procedures must describe the distribution process for each drug. This includes procedures for recalls.
4. Written procedures must describe the appropriate storage conditions for each drug.

A major pharmaceutical warehousing challenge involves these "appropriate storage conditions." Different drugs can have vastly different requirements in terms of temperature, humidity, and lighting. The warehousing provider must ensure that the storage of each drug is in line with its specific requirements defined by the manufacturer. This can involve **temperature-controlled warehousing** and/or **climate-controlled warehousing space** – both of which require state-of-the-art control and monitoring equipment to keep the space within specific environmental parameters.

(i) Temperature-controlled space requires sophisticated control and monitoring equipment to ensure that the temperature of the facility stays within very specific parameters.

(ii) Climate-controlled space regulates and monitors both the temperature and humidity of the space.

Selecting a Warehousing Partner

When looking for a logistics provider to handle a pharmaceutical warehousing operation, there are plenty of things to look for. In addition to the cGMPs listed above, a prospective logistics partner should be able to demonstrate the following:

1. The facility should be clean and have adequate space for storage that also allows for maintenance, and inspection. It should have adequate lighting, ventilation, and environmental conditions for the drugs being stored. There should also be a quarantine area for drugs that have expired or otherwise can no longer be used.
2. The facility's security systems and processes – both inside and outside – must be able to prevent unauthorized entry and protect against theft.
3. Drugs without specific storage requirements should be stored at "controlled room temperature" (according to the FDA).
4. The provider's inventory and WMS systems must be able to provide visibility into product location.
5. The logistics partner must be able to provide written documentation of policies and procedures as well as inventories and distribution.

Kanban Logistics for Pharmaceutical Warehousing

Very few logistics providers are available for pharmaceutical products. Kanban (Kanban's pharmaceutical industry solutions) is one such logistic provider.

Kanban is registered with the FDA and adheres to all CGMP regulations and voluntarily undergoes audits from the FDA and from new clients during the on boarding process. Kanban is also ISO-9001:2015-certified which allows consistently deliver quality to the customers, while continually optimizing performance across the board.

Materials Management

Materials management involves planning, programming, organizing, directing, controlling, and coordinating the various activities concerning the materials. The production managers found it necessary to develop an organized body of knowledge on this subject. The resulting set of related disciplines is known as materials management. Materials are any commodities used directly or indirectly in producing a product such as raw materials, component parts or assemblies. Materials management is the grouping of management functions supporting the complete cycle of material flow, from the purchase and internal control of production materials to the planning and control of work in process to the warehousing, shipping, and distribution of the finished product. Materials management is the management of the flow of materials into an organization to the point, where, those materials are converted into the firm's end product(s).

Basic Activities of Materials Management

The executives who engage in materials management are concerned with three basic activities:

Buying

Storage of materials and

- Movement of materials

Functions of Materials Management

The following are the functions of material managements.

1. Materials planning and programming
2. Raw material purchase
3. Receiving, store keeping, and warehousing
4. Issuing of material
5. Inventory control
6. Value engineering
7. Transportation of materials
8. Vendor development
9. Vendor rating
10. Disposal of scrap and surpluses

Focus of Material Management is to procure to procure right materials in right quantity, of right quality, at right time, from right sources and at right prices. These 5 R's are principles of purchasing.

The Objectives of Materials Management

The primary objectives of materials management include buying the best item at the lowest cost, reduction in inventory cost and high inventory turnover, maintaining the flow of production, maintaining the consistency of quality, optimization of acquisition and possession, resulting in lower cost, cordial relationship with suppliers, maintaining good records, contribution towards competitiveness, and personnel development.

The secondary objectives of materials management include, promotion of standardization with suppliers, development of reciprocal relations with customers, committees to decide on economic make or buy decisions, development of inter departmental relationships and can undertake acquisitions.

Advantages or Benefits of Materials Management

The following are the advantages/ benefits of material management

1. Material cost can be lowered (Sales price can be brought down to a reasonable level)
2. Controlling of indirect cost (such as materials movement)
3. Risk of inventory loss minimized (theft, pilferage)
4. Reduction in loss of time of direct labor
5. Cost of material used in different department ascertained
6. Control of manufacturing cycle
7. Material congestion in storage places avoided
8. Improvement in delivery of the product

Stages of Material Management

1. Planning (Plans for capacity or production levels and required inventory levels)
2. Material utilization (efficiency of the flow of materials through the plant)
3. Physical (storing, receiving and issuing of materials and physical checking of inventory of raw materials, work in process, finished goods, record keeping)
4. Control or follow up (feedback and corrective action involved)

Challenges of Material Management

The challenges of material management include Selection of appropriate vendors; Land and storage cost increase; Difficulty in forecasting demand accurately; Scarce capital for investment in materials inventory; Diversification of product lines; Optimizing time and quantity for products and Management of information.

Organization of Material Management

Material management consist of following four main departments/ activities

1. Materials planning;
2. Purchase;
3. Stores;
4. Inventory control

Purchasing

- Purchasing is to procure the materials, supplies, tools, equipment etc.
- The principles of 5 R's (as described earlier) shall be used for procuring materials.

Importance of Purchasing

1. Purchasing function provides materials to the factory without which the machines cannot move.
2. A one percent saving in cost is equivalent to 10 percent increase in turnover
3. Purchasing manager is the custodian of his firm's purse as he spends more than 50% of his company's earnings on purchases
4. Increasing proportion of one's requirements are now bought instead of being made.
5. Can contribute to import substitution and can save foreign exchange
6. Purchasing is the main contributor for the timely execution of industrial projects
7. Materials management organizations that exist now have evolved out of purchasing departments.
8. Other factors- cyclical swings of surpluses and shortages and the fast rising material costs, heavy competition, growing worldwide markets have contributed to the importance of purchasing

Objectives of Purchasing

The following are the objectives of purchasing

1. Procurement of required quantity and quality of materials at the most economical price
2. Procuring the material well in advance to meet the needs of the production dept, to save production losses from lack of materials
3. Buying an optimum quantity, neither too much nor too less, not affecting capital or holding up production.
4. Improvement of the product with reference to quality by means of selection of adequate material.
5. To keep top management aware of costs involved in the company's procurement and any market change that would affect the company's profit or growth potential.
6. To develop fullest cooperation, coordination and maintenance of internal relationship with departments in the company.

7. To initiate, if necessary, and cooperate in cost reduction programmes, value analysis, make or buy decisions, market analysis and long range planning. Purchasing should keep abreast with trends and projections in prices and the availability of the inputs that a company must have.

Purchasing Cycle

1. Recognition of need
2. Description of need
3. A suitable source is selected.
4. Often a source has to be developed.
5. Price and availability are determined.
6. Purchase order is prepared and sent to the supplier
7. Acceptance of the purchase order is obtained from the supplier
8. Follow up is done by the purchase dept. to ensure timely delivery of the material.
9. Checking the invoice and approving it for making payment to the supplier

Categories of purchasing needs:

1. Low volume, infrequent purchase of small monetary value
2. One-time infrequent purchase of significant monetary value
3. High volume purchases used over time or in multiple locations

Vendor rating

Vendor rating is a method to evaluate a vendor against certain parameters, related to his supplies.

The following factors are to be considered for vendor rating:

1. Vendors are assessed on the basis of a wide variety of factors or criteria which might include but not limited to: Price, Discounts received, Maintenance of specifications.
2. Promptness of delivery
3. Freight and delivery charges
4. Service
5. Market information
6. Cooperation
7. Management competence
8. Credit terms
9. Cost reduction suggestions

10. Inventory plans
11. Financial position

Rating Techniques

1. **Categorical plan**

   Personnel from different division maintain informal evaluation records, Purchasing, engineering, quality control, receiving and inspection, For each supplier, each person prepares a list of performance factors important to him. At a monthly meeting, each major supplier is evaluated against the list and assigned an overall group evaluation, like "preferred", "neutral", or "unsatisfactory".

2. **Weighted point plan**

   The performance factors to be evaluated are given "weights", for example quality might be weighted 25, delivery 20, price 30 and service 25. Weights selected represent buyer's judgment about the relative importance of the respective factors. (Quantitative terms)

3. **Critical incidents method**

   Record of events related to buyer vendor relationships is maintained in each vendor's file. They reflect positive and negative aspect of actual performance. This kind of documentation useful in discussing ways and means of improving performance, acknowledging the existence of good relationships, determining the competence of a vendor, and if necessary considering termination.

4. **Checklist system**

   A simple checklist is used to evaluate the vendors. Check list may be something like Reliability, technical capability, after sales service, availability, buying convenience etc.

Ethics

- Ethics is a segment of philosophy concerned with values of human conduct.
- Ethics refers to a code of conduct that guides an individual in dealing with others.
- Ethics relates to the social rules that influence people to be honest in dealing with others.

Ethics in Purchasing

Many decisions remain largely a matter of personal judgement. Purchase manager is the custodian of company funds, responsible for their conservation and wise spending. Because of his contacts, he is the custodian of company's reputation for courtesy and fair dealing. A high ethical standard of conduct is essential. They are subjected to more temptations. Since they spend millions, they yield tremendous power and are the objects of considerable attention from suppliers. They are in an excellent position to be dishonest if they want to. But they have to be ethical.

Value Analysis (Value Engineering)

Purchasing & methods engineering. This activity is aimed at modifying the specifications of materials, parts, and products to reduce their costs. Focus is on the value of the product- what function is to be performed by the product and how that value can be achieved at the lowest cost. Primary attention is devoted to the materials. Suppliers suggest improvement & cost reduction ideas.

Inventory Management

- The term inventory includes materials raw, in process, finished packaging, spares and others stocked in order to meet an unexpected demand or distribution in the future.
- Inventory can be used to refer to the stock on hand at a particular time, of raw materials, goods-in-process of manufacture, finished products, and merchandise purchased for resale, and the like, tangible assets which can be seen, measured and counted. In connection with financial statements and accounting records, the reference may be to the amount assigned to the stock of goods owned by an enterprise at a particular time.

Types of Inventories

- Finished goods inventories
- Stock in trade, ready for shipment
- Maintenance, Repair and Operating inventories
- -cutting tools, grinding wheels, jigs
- Maintenance inventory
- Electrical, switches, fuses, lamps, lubricants, safety goggles
- Stationary inventories
- Canteen provisions, medical supplies, uniforms

Objectives of Inventory

1. To facilitate smooth operation of the manufacturing process.
2. To minimize investment in inventory
3. To reduce material handling costs

4. Reasonable utilization of people
5. Inventories are held to facilitate product display and service to customers, batching in production in order to take advantage of longer production runs and provide flexibility in production scheduling.

Benefits of Inventory Management

1. Inventory control ensures an adequate supply of materials, stores, etc. minimizes stock outs and shortages, and avoids costly interruptions in operations.
2. It keeps down investments in inventories, inventory carrying costs and obsolescence losses to the minimum.
3. It facilitates purchasing economies through the measurement of requirements on the basis of recorded experience
4. It eliminates duplication in ordering or in replenishing stocks by centralizing the source from which purchase requisitions emanate
5. It permits a better utilization of available stocks by facilitating inter departmental transfers within a company
6. It provides a check against loss of materials through carelessness or pilferage
7. It facilitates cost accounting activities by providing a means for allocating material costs to products, departments or other operating accounts
8. It enables management to make cost and consumption comparison between operations and periods.
9. It serves as a means for the location and disposition of inactive and obsolete items of stores.
10. Perpetual inventory values provide a consistent and reliable basis for preparing financial statements.

Printed by Libri Plureos GmbH in Hamburg,
Germany

9 789389 354966